Smart and Secure Internet of Healthcare Things

Internet of Healthcare Things (IoHT) is an Internet of Things (IoT)-based solution that includes a network architecture which allows the connection between a patient and healthcare facilities. This book covers various research issues of smart and secure IoHT, aimed at providing solutions for remote healthcare monitoring using pertinent techniques. Applications of machine learning techniques and data analytics in IoHT, along with the latest communication and networking technologies and cloud computing, are also discussed.

Features:

- Provides a detailed introduction to IoHT and its applications
- Reviews underlying sensor and hardware technologies
- Includes recent advances in the IoHT, such as remote healthcare monitoring and wearable devices
- Explores applications of data analytics/data mining in IoHT, including data management and data governance
- Focuses on regulatory and compliance issues in IoHT

This book is intended for graduate students and researchers in Bioinformatics, Biomedical Engineering, Big Data and Analytics, Data Mining, and Information Management, IoT and Computer and Electrical Engineering.

Advances in Smart Healthcare Technologies

Series Editors: *Chinmay Chakraborty and Joel J. P. C. Rodrigues*

Series Description:
This book series focus on recent advances and different research areas in smart healthcare technologies including Internet of Medical Things (IoMedT), e-Health, personalized medicine, sensing, Big data, telemedicine, etc. under the healthcare informatics umbrella. Overall focus is on bringing together the latest industrial and academic progress, research and development efforts within the rapidly maturing health informatics ecosystem. It aims to offer valuable perceptions to researchers and engineers on how to design and develop novel healthcare systems and how to improve patient's information delivery care remotely. The potential for making faster advances in many scientific disciplines and improving the profitability and success of different enterprises is to be investigated.

Blockchain Technology in Healthcare Applications: Social, Economic and Technological Implications
Bharat Bhushan, Nitin Rakesh, Yousef Farhaoui, Parma Nand Astya and Bhuvan Unhelkar

Digital Health Transformation with Blockchain and Artificial Intelligence
Chinmay Chakraborty

Smart and Secure Internet of Healthcare Things
Nitin Gupta, Jagdeep Singh, Chinmay Chakraborty, Mamoun Alazab and Dinh-Thuan Do

For more information, please visit: https://www.routledge.com/Advances-in-Smart-Healthcare-Technologies/book-series/CRCASHT

Smart and Secure Internet of Healthcare Things

Edited by

Nitin Gupta

Jagdeep Singh

Chinmay Chakraborty

Mamoun Alazab

Dinh-Thuan Do

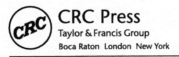

CRC Press
Taylor & Francis Group
Boca Raton London New York

CRC Press is an imprint of the
Taylor & Francis Group, an **informa** business

First edition published 2023
by CRC Press
6000 Broken Sound Parkway NW, Suite 300, Boca Raton, FL 33487-2742

and by CRC Press
4 Park Square, Milton Park, Abingdon, Oxon, OX14 4RN

CRC Press is an imprint of Taylor & Francis Group, LLC

ISBN: 978-1-032-14549-5 (hbk)
ISBN: 978-1-032-14550-1 (pbk)
ISBN: 978-1-003-23989-5 (ebk)

DOI: 10.1201/9781003239895

Typeset in Nimbus font
by KnowledgeWorks Global Ltd.

Contents

Preface

The Internet of Things (IoT) is going to impact the healthcare system in a big way. IoT-Based solutions that include a network architecture that allows the connection between a patient and healthcare facilities is termed as the Internet of Healthcare Things (IoHT) or Internet of Medical Things (IoMT). IoHT can be used to monitor the patients located in far areas. Various types of monitoring like ECG and diabetes can be done through IoHT. Various major hospitals also send digital CT scan reports to a cloud system for processing using IoHT. Moreover, a large amount of patient data is routinely manually collected in hospitals by using stand-alone medical devices, including vital signs. Such data is sometimes stored in spreadsheets, not forming part of patients' electronic health records, and is therefore difficult for caregivers to combine and analyse. One possible solution to overcome these limitations is the interconnection of medical devices via IoHT. Therefore, IoHT provides the solution to many problems that otherwise are difficult to solve manually. The book provides the latest research areas and concepts in the proposed subject. Various practical applications and case studies are covered in this book which will create an interest among readers. This book will help readers grasp the latest viewpoint and the quintessence of the recent advances that are happening around the world in this area. A brief introduction about each chapter is as follows:

Chapter 1 briefs on the various healthcare solutions using wearable devices. Examples of various wearable devices used to monitor remote patients and used in sports and animal tracking are also provided. Chapter 2 discusses various disease prediction strategies using IoHT. Further, the detailed literature review of various disease predictions, like Alzheimer's, that is done is explored. Chapter 3 discusses posture detection of a patient using IoHT. The chapter explores underlying sensors and their technology that can be considered for posture and fall detection of elderly patients.

Chapters 4 and 5 introduce the concept and applications of artificial intelligence and machine learning in the field of IoHT. Various case studies focusing on their applications in IoHT have also been discussed.

Chapters 6, 7 and 8 touch on the aspects of various security and privacy concerns that can arise in the IoHT domain. Various countermeasures and research challenges are discussed, which will help the researchers working in security-related areas to explore the promising IoHT field.

Chapter 9 explores the future wireless communication techniques like cloud/edge computing, etc., that will play an important role in enabling future IoMT services and applications, and Chapter 10 discusses an energy-efficient routing and aggregation protocol for Wireless body area networks that can play a big part in IoHT.

Lastly, Chapter 11 sums up the book by introducing very important case studies of some of the countries of the world that successfully implemented the IoHT network to handle various recent epidemics and pandemics. This chapter will give an idea to the researchers on how they can proceed with the implementation of IoHT in their own country also.

The editors are thankful to the authors and reviewers for their excellent contributions in making this book possible. Our special thanks to Prof. Joel J. P. C. Rodrigues and Dr. Chinmay Chakraborty (series editors) for giving us the opportunity to edit the book. We would also like to thank Dr. Gagandeep Singh and Ms. Aditi Mittal, CRC Press, who coordinated the entire proceedings. We hope that the book will be useful to a wide variety of readers and will provide useful insight to all.

Nitin Gupta
Jagdeep Singh
Chinmay Chakraborty
Mamoun Alazab
Dinh-Thuan Do

Editors

Dr. Nitin Gupta has served as an Assistant Professor with the Department of Computer Science and Engineering, NIT Hamirpur, Himachal Pradesh, India since 2007. He received his PhD degree from NSIT, University of Delhi under the supervision of Prof. Sanjay Kumar Dhurandher. His research interest includes efficient resource allocation in Next Generation Wireless Networks, especially Cognitive Radio Networks. He has published various research papers in High-Impact reputed international journals like *IEEE Transactions on Vehicular Technology, IEEE TNSE* and *IEEE Systems Journal* and conferences of repute like IEEE ICC, GLOBECOM and INFOCOM. He is an IEEE Senior Member, member of the IEEE Communication Society and member of the ACM as well. He is also a member of the Executive Committee of the IEEE Communication Society, Delhi Chapter. Currently, he is also serving as an Associate Editor in IEEE Access & IJSNet, Inderscience and earlier served as a Guest Editor in IEEE TGCN, ETT, Wiley, SUSCOM Elsevier and others. Along with organizing various short-term courses and conferences, he was also a member of technical program committees of various IEEE/ACM/Springer/Scopus conferences. He is a reviewer of various reputed journals like *IEEE Transactions on Wireless Communications, IEEE Transactions on Industrial Informatics, IEEE Systems Journal* and *IJCS Wiley.*

Dr. Jagdeep Singh received his PhD degree in Computer Engineering from the University of Delhi, New Delhi, India. Currently, he is working as an Assistant Professor in the Department of Computer Science Engineering, Sant Longowal Institute of Engineering & Technology (SLIET), Longowal. His current research interests include Wireless Networks, Network Security, Reinforcement Learning and Artificial Intelligence. He has published research papers in very highly reputed journals like *IEEE Internet of Things, Journal of Ambient Intelligence and Humanized Computing, IET* and *International Journal of Communication Systems*. He has also presented his research work in several international flagship conferences, such as IEEE ICC, IEEE Globecom and AINA.

Dr. Chinmay Chakraborty, SMIEEE is an Assistant Professor in Electronics and Communication Engineering, Birla Institute of Technology, Mesra, India, and he completed his Post-doctoral fellowship from Federal University of Piauí, Brazil. His main research interests include the Internet of Medical Things, Wireless Body Sensor Networks, Wireless Networks, Telemedicine, m-Health/e-health and Medical Imaging. He received a Best Session Runner-up Award, Young Research Excellence Award, Global Peer Review Award, Young Faculty Award, Outstanding Researcher Award and was also selected as one of the top 2% of scientists in the world in the field of 'Artificial Intelligence and Image Processing', Stanford University, USA.

Mamoun Alazab is an Associate Professor at the College of Engineering, IT and Environment at Charles Darwin University, Australia. He received his PhD degree in Computer Science from the Federation University of Australia, School of Science, Information Technology and Engineering. He is the recipient of the prestigious award, NT Young Tall Poppy (2021) of the year from the Australian Institute of Policy and Science (AIPS), and the Japan Society for the Promotion of Science (JSPS) fellowship through the Australian Academy of Science. He worked previously as a Senior Lecturer (Australian National University) and Lecturer (Macquarie University). He is a cyber-security researcher and practitioner with industry and academic experience. Associate Prof. Alazab's research is multidisciplinary and focuses on cyber security with a focus on cybercrime detection and prevention. He has more than 300 research papers (>90% in Q1 and in the top 10% of journal articles, and more than 100 in IEEE/ACM Transactions) and 11 authored/edited books. He is a Senior Member of the IEEE, and the founding chair of the IEEE Northern Territory (NT) Subsection. He serves as the Associate Editor of *IEEE Transactions on Computational Social Systems*, *IEEE Transactions on Network and Service Management (TNSM)*, *IEEE Internet of Things Journal*, *ACM Digital Threats: Research and Practice* and *Complex & Intelligent Systems*.

Dinh-Thuan Do (Senior Member, IEEE) received the BS, MEng and PhD degrees from Vietnam National University (VNU-HCMC) in 2003, 2007 and 2013, respectively, all in communications engineering. Prior to joining University of Colorado, Denver (USA), he also worked with the University of Texas at Austin (USA), Asia University (Taiwan) and Ton Duc Thang University (Vietnam). His research interests include signal processing in wireless communications networks, non-orthogonal multiple access, full-duplex transmission, machine learning for wireless networks and reconfigurable intelligent surfaces (RIS). Dr. Thuan was a recipient of the Golden Globe Award from the Vietnam Ministry of Science and Technology in 2015 (top ten excellent scientists nationwide). He is currently serving as an Editor of IEEE *Trans. On Vehicular Technology*, *Computer Communications* (Elsevier), EURASIP *Journal on Wireless Communications and Networking* (Springer), *ICT Express* and *KSII Transactions on Internet and Information Systems*. His publications include over 100 SCIE/SCI-indexed journal articles, and over 50 international conference papers. He is the sole author of one textbook, one edited book and eight book chapters.

Contributors

Ahed Abugabah
Zayed University
United Arab Emirates

Subhrangshu Adhikary
Dr. B.C. Roy Engineering College
Durgapur, India

Idoia Aguirre
Centro de Innovación Tecnológica
de Automoción de Nevarro
NAITEC
Spain

Omar Alfandi
Zayed University
United Arab Emirates

José Javier Astrain
Universidad Pública de Navarra
and Institute for Smart Cities
(ISC)-UPNA
Spain

Summit Bandotra
Lovely Professional University
Phagwara, Punjab, India

Jagadeesha R Bhat
Indian Institute of Information
Technology, Dharwad
Karnataka, India

Amartya Chakraborty
University of Engineering and
Management
Kolkata, India

Jesús Daniel Trigo
Universidad Pública de Navarra and
Institute for Smart Cities
(ISC)-UPNA
Spain

Pankaj Dhiman
Jaypee University of Information
Technology
Solan, Himachal Pradesh, India

Ritwik Duggal
National Institute of Technology
Hamirpur, Himachal Pradesh, India

Ramya Elango
Bannari Amman Inst. of Tech.
Sathyamangalam, India

Francisco Falcone
Universidad Pública de Navarra and
Institute for Smart Cities
(ISC)-UPNA
Spain

Pranjal Garg
All India Institute of Medical Science
Rishikesh, Uttrakhand, India

Arindam Ghosh
Dr. B.C. Roy Engineering College
Durgapur, India

Jahnvi Gupta
National Institute of Technology
Hamirpur, Himachal Pradesh, India

Nitin Gupta
National Institute of Technology
Hamirpur, Himachal Pradesh, India

Sejal Gupta
National Institute of Technology
Kurukshetra, Haryana, India

Abinaya Inbamani
Sri Ramakrishna Engineering College
Coimbatore, India

Deepa Krishnan
Mukesh Patel School of Technology,
    Management, and Engineering,
    NMIMS University
Mumbai, Maharashtra, India

Mukesh Kumar
National Institute of Technology
Hamirpur, Himachal Pradesh, India

Rakesh Kumar
Central University of Haryana
Mahendargarh, India

Rakesh Kumar Jha
PDPM Indian Institute of Information
    Technology Design and
    Manufacturing
Jabalpur, Madhya Pradesh, India

Manu.V.T.
Vel Tech Rangarajan Dr.Sagunthala
    R&D Institute of Science and
    Technology
Chennai, Tamil Nadu, India

S. Niveda
Sri Ramakrishna Engineering College
Coimbatore, India

M. Preethi
Sri Ramakrishna Engineering College
Coimbatore, India

R. Rajalakshmi
Sri Ramakrishna Engineering College
Coimbatore, India

Roopali Punj
National Institute of Technical Teachers
    Training and Research
Chandigarh, India

A. Siva Sakthi
Sri Ramakrishna Engineering College
Coimbatore, India

Partha Sarathi Paul
Indian Institute of Technology
Kharagpur, India

Luis Serrano
Universidad Pública de Navarra and
    Institute for Smart Cities
    (ISC)-UPNA
Spain

Misbah Shafi
Shri Mata Vaishno Devi University
Katra, Jammu and Kashmir, India

Jang-Ping Sheu
National Tsing Hua University
Hsinchu, Taiwan

Swapnil Singh
Mukesh Patel School of Technology,
    Management, and Engineering,
    NMIMS University
Mumbai, Maharashtra, India

Sitara K.
National Institute of Technology
Tiruchirappalli, Tamil Nadu, India

Ankit Songara
PwC Bangalore
Karnataka, India

Veerapandiyan Veerasamy
University Putra
Malaysia

1 Healthcare Solutions Using Wearable Devices

A. Siva Sakthi, Abinaya Inbamani, Ramya Elango,
S. Niveda, M. Preethi, R. Rajalakshmi and
Veerapandiyan Veerasamy

CONTENTS

1.1 INTRODUCTION

With advancements in science and technology, the miniaturization of electronic components plays a vital role in numerous fields; one such is the customization of medical devices into wearable devices. Wearable medical devices have been used in every aspect of daily living. They have their unique place in the medical world to

DOI: 10.1201/9781003239895-1

monitor patients remotely. They also find applications in sports medicine, animal tracking and activity monitoring. Nowadays wearable devices like fitness bands are more preferred by almost all kind of people to monitor their health. They use wearable technology which is further classified into two parts, the wearable and body sensor. The wearable is defined as anything that can be worn by the user, whereas body sensor is placed on the human body to acquire various physical parameters like blood pressure, temperature, pH, etc. Body sensors include accelerometer, gyroscopes, temperature sensor, etc. Wearable devices are mainly preferred because of their comfort, non-invasiness and aesthetic appearance. They can perform particular medical function, either as a supporting device or as a monitoring device for prolonged time period. Internet of Things (IoT) plays a major role in wearable technology, with life-changing applications in medicine and also in other fields. Wearable medical devices are socially acceptable for their design. They can be worn as a wrist watch, rings, shoes, ear buds and even in the form of textiles. Textile-based wearable devices are evolving in this digital world as they are more pleasing and comfortable. A user can wear such devices and be stress-free as wearable devices function on their own.

Wearable devices help to monitor a person's health in various aspects, by measuring blood pressure, heart rate, Parkinson's and tremor, breathing patterns, diet, stroke, cancer, diabetes, respiratory rate and various physiological parameters like electrocardiogram (ECG), electromyogram (EMG), temperature, pH, etc. The basic wearable device contains a sensor, a radio frequency (RF) module, a microcontroller unit (MCU) board, a battery and a power management unit. As an example, a wearable device for monitoring the intake of solid and liquid foods is available in the form of a necklace. This necklace measures the volume of food consumption and transmits data to the user with the help of a mobile application, which is integrated with IoT [1]. The various wearable devices available in the market are depicted in Figure 1.1.

1.2 VARIOUS SENSORS AND TECHNOLOGY USED TO DEVELOP A WEARABLE DEVICE LIKE IOT

The objective of the sensor is to collect data from the environment that helps to convert physical variables into electrical signals. IoT means connecting the things that consist of sensors, microcontrollers and transceivers to the internet. IoT devices share the collected data from the sensor and communicate the information over the network without human interaction. Hence it is called as machine-to-machine communication. Sensor is the major component in developing any wearable device. The sensors used in wearable technology are broadly classified as biomechanical sensors and physiological sensors. Biomechanical sensors are used to measure motions and vibrations in the region of interest. It consists of accelerometers, gyroscopes, inertial sensors and so on. Physiological sensors are used to acquire physiological parameters such as temperature, pressure, pH and also electrical activity of the heart, brain, muscles, etc. Some examples for this sensor include electrodes, piezoelectric sensors, piezoresistive sensors, biochemical sensors, gas sensors, etc.

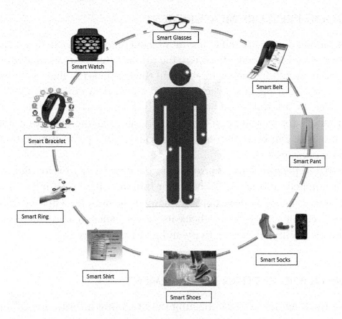

Figure 1.1 Various wearable devices

For wearable electronics, direct patterning flexible circuits can be designed. On a nylon fabric, Cu electroless deposition (ELD) is ink jetted. To the fabric, a chitosan solution is coated prior to the printing of $AgNO_3$, which results in good stability and flexibility. To create electronic textiles, direct metallization approach is used [2]. Applications of various sensors are summarized in Figure 1.2.

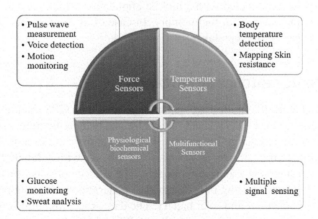

Figure 1.2 Sensors and their applications

1.2.1 BLOOD PRESSURE MEASUREMENT

A finger-wearable device is used to monitor blood pressure, consisting of a capacitive tactile sensor which is placed adjacent to the digital artery. An air bladder driven by a pump is used to sweep the pressure, wherein the tactile array that contacts the finger is being pressed. During this sweep, the waveform data collected from the digital artery provides the arterial blood pressure. This device performs better with the lasso regression model for systolic and diastolic pressure. Using such wearable devices, the blood pressure can be monitored continuously, thus preventing fatality rate due to high blood pressure [3].

Textile-based piezoresistive sensors were designed using highly flexible conductive threads stitched onto fabric. This sensor monitors the breathing rate through rib cage, and step counting is done through hamstring muscle. This wearable cloth is machine washed for ten cycles to check its performance. The result shows high response time, flexibility, high sensitivity and good reliability [4].

1.2.2 BREATHING PATTERN MEASUREMENT

A wearable tracking device for collecting the breathing information of a patient has also been proposed [5]. It consists of a differential pressure sensor attached with the face mask, and the gas flow rate is obtained by estimating the difference in pressure produced by the orifice passage. The face mask uses two separate channels for inhalation and exhalation during breathing. In the breathing flow measurement module, dynamic tracking and signal compensation algorithms are executed [5].

A wearable cloth for monitoring chronic breathing problems is implemented in [6]. The smart clothing helps to monitor various disorders like sleep apnoea, cough, asthma and sneezing all the time. The components are mended on the cloth and charged using a battery. It consists of a flex sensor, embedded in the shirt. It continuously monitors the breathing rate and the expansion and contraction of the abdomen. It is interconnected with a mobile application which records the patient's breathing rate and stores it in the memory. In case of any emergencies, it sends an immediate message to the caretaker.

1.2.3 AUTISTIC CHILDREN MONITORING

A smart wearable health monitoring technology along with GPS tracking can be used to monitor autistic children [7]. Heart rate, pulse and body temperature of the autistic children are monitored using this device. When the autistic children go outside, parents will be able to track the location on a regular basis, with a detailed notification. It also provides emergency alert immediately. The device consists of a power generation unit and data processing unit. The power generation unit contains a miniature solar cell, boost converter and solar battery. The data processing unit contains a pulse sensor, temperature sensor, microcontroller, GPS and GSM module and emergency button.

1.2.4 TEMPERATURE MONITORING

A wearable device to measure the temperature, ultraviolet (UV) index under sunlight and the level of skin hydration was presented by Yang et al. to avoid skin cancer [8]. The device looks like a smart bracelet or ring which estimates the skin hydration due to sunlight exposure. It contains communication interfaces and impedance channel with copper electrodes. It uses near field communication (NFC) interface to calculate the UV index using the energy harvested from the mobile phone. With the help of this device, early diagnosis of skin cancer is possible.

1.2.5 MONITORING OF ELDERLY PEOPLE

Wearable devices can also be used to monitor the physical activity of elderly people and can remind them to take medications at the appropriate time [9]. It consists of a set of sensors, an accelerometer, a gyroscope and a heartbeat detector. The device is a small and lightweight design which is worn on the chest to sense their movements. An SD card is used to store the physical activity data. The postural movements are captured by the accelerometer and gyroscope. An irregular sign of the movements and fall of the patients is detected and recorded by the on-board microcontroller.

1.2.6 MEDICATION MONITORING

Wearable sensors are available to measure medication and physiological signals. It consists of an ingestible sensor placed in the patient's stomach, and a wearable unit is placed on the patient's skin. The ingestible sensor gets associated with gastric fluids, and the information collected is communicated to the wearable sensor or patch. The wearable unit contains a low-noise amplifier, power circuits, LEDs, an accelerometer, a temperature sensor, a SoC, a Bluetooth radio and a flash memory. The patch is a body-worn device which measures various parameters like heart rate, body angle and step count [10].

To view the movement disorders, a novel textile-embedded low-power wearable device is used. The iHandU performs rigid changes in Parkinson's disease-based patients during deep brain stimulation (DBS) surgeries. The device is placed around the patient's hand, and gyroscope data is transmitted to an android application score for the rigidity change [11].

1.2.7 FERTILITY MONITORING

Fertility awareness is the need of the hour to make sexual and reproductive decisions among couples. The pattern of ovulation duration can be observed using a wearable device [12]. This can be done by measuring the abdominal thickness and basal body temperature. It consists of a flex sensor or bend sensor which is used to compute the thickness of the abdomen (mm), and to measure the temperature of the body, DS 18B20 is used. This device has two competencies. Firstly, the data is passed securely to the doctor. Secondly, the ovulation week is predicted. This obtained data is sent cryptographically using the algorithms such as deoxyribonucleic acid (DNA) and HUFFMAN. Hence, machine learning techniques like support vector machine (SVM) provides good accuracy for tracking the ovulation.

1.2.8 WEARABLE GLASS

A wearable glass for visually impaired people has been developed with the help of IoT and computer vision [13]. It consists of a built-in bone conduction and microphone unit, an object recognition module, face recognition, and a processing unit which communicates via Bluetooth. It also helps to navigate blind people. Through bone conduction technology, the glass can visualize the surroundings, take in commands and send information to the wearer which helps to connect them with the surrounding real-time environment. This device helps blind people by guiding them to cross the obstacle. Various types of sensors and their applications are listed in Table 1.1.

1.3 WEARABLE DEVICE TO MONITOR REMOTE PATIENTS FOR BETTER DIAGNOSIS AND TREATMENT

Many wearable healthcare innovation technology applications range from checking daily tasks to assess strength, quality and the level of independence in people, by incorporating tiny sensors into gadgets and clothing to reinforce the technologies that assist patients in performing various useful motor tasks that they can't do independently, i.e. without the help of family or caretaker. These technologies can monitor physical activity, hypertension/hypotension, core body temperature, blood glucose level and heart and brain activity remotely. Given the flexibility of those devices to provide feedback on health and physiological status of each person and then enable medical care professionals to optimize treatment choices based on the feedback, this collected information is usually used for diagnostic purposes. It is also used to work out the restoration development of an individual recovering from an associate injury or illness, given the flexibility of those devices to supply feedback on health and physiological status for each person and then enable medical care professionals to optimize treatment choices based on the information [21].

The wearable clinical electronic gadgets can measure different health indicators. For example, pulse rate, heart rate, core body temperature, blood glucose and so on non-invasively by basically attaching them to the human body surface. Constant observing of vital signs can help the individuals and healthcare providers, an additional clinical consideration when a person's actual physical healthcare markers are unusual, keeping away from the circumstance where the best therapy time is missed. Likewise, adaptable hardware can be distorted voluntarily and identify different sensors with amazingly high sensitivity; this can be utilized in various modes like artificial electronic skin, movement detection, telemedicine and in-home medical care. There is no uncertainty that next-generation adaptable and wearable gadgets will prompt a transformation in the human lifestyle. Furthermore, as remote patients are prompt to innovation technology, then it turns out to be more intelligent and more reasonable for the invention of new electronic gadgets in the market. This can

Table 1.1

Various Types of Wearable Sensors and Their Applications

Reference	Type of Sensor Used	Application	Location on Body
Presti et al. [14]	Fibre Bragg grating (FBG) sensor	Monitoring of cardiac activity	Chest
Sriraam.N et al. [15]	Electrodes for bio potential monitoring [SiPNyW (Silver-plated nylon-woven)-based textile electrode belt with lead-I configuration]	Recording of ECG signal	Chest
Saied et al. [16]	RF sensors for detecting changes in the brain	Detects the progression of brain atrophy and lateral ventricle enlargement in patients with Alzheimer's	Head
Kostikis et al. [17]	Accelerometers and/or gyroscopes	To monitor Parkinson's disease (PD) symptoms	Wristbands and a necklace
Fadhillah et al. [18]	Thermal sensors and thermal imaging camera	Breast cancer monitoring	Thermal sensors positioned on brassiere cloth covering all four quadrants
Sasidharan et al. [19]	Embedded garment sensor	Foetal movement monitoring	Abdomen
Jeon et al. [20]	PAAR band and Biocradle	Sleep disorders	Wristwatch

be accessed by an emergency clinic with an intend to give new potential profit channels [22].

1.3.1 BENEFITS OF REMOTE PATIENT MONITORING DEVICES

Remote patient monitoring gadgets are getting more and more popular because of the level of trust and transparency they provide. The innovation permits suppliers to have a more profound understanding of the patient condition who is suffering from decision-making in selecting the available choices of treatment. Remote monitoring gadgets have surely reduced expenses while focusing on comfort and suitability for the patients and service providers. It saved time and costs due to long-distance travel. It also plays a major role in saving patients' time and energy to recover. It can also reduce pressure and tension for patients who have financial hindrances to get an effective treatment protocol.

1.3.2 FUNCTION MODULES OF REMOTE PATIENT MONITORING DEVICES

Wearable devices use IoT-Based remote patient health monitoring system. The improved and intellectual medical structure is an image of an established and wealthy country. The IoT has boosted the digital medical structure by allowing remote monitoring of patients' medical conditions and helps in accessing the data by medical specialists remotely [23].

IoT-Based automatic and intelligent framework detects patients' medical difficulties originally, stores and displays that information over the internet and alerts medical specialists over critical situations. The wearable device would keep doctors updated about their patients' health issues continuously. In case of emergency, it will notify both the doctor and the caretaker about the patient's status. As a result, the percentage of lives saved will get increased, and a doctor will be able to provide medical treatment and advise to a larger number of individuals in a shorter period of time due to remote monitoring.

The IoT-Based remote monitoring framework has two sides: one at the web application, which includes the database, and the other at the user-end, which includes a wearable sensor. The system block diagram of the IoT devices considered in the framework is depicted in Figure 1.3.

The piezoelectric sensor collects the physiological signals from the user, whereas the temperature sensor collects the temperature profile and is fed to the microcontroller for processing. This data is fed to the server via a Wi-Fi module. LM35 provides the patient's continual body temperature. Since, it is in direct contact with the patient, the temperature sensor is placed beneath the device for the greatest results. Further, every ten minutes, the microcontroller collects data from the sensors and communicates it to the server using a SIM 900D GSM module. In the event of an adverse situation, microcontroller sends an SMS to the crisis contact through GSM SIM900D [23].

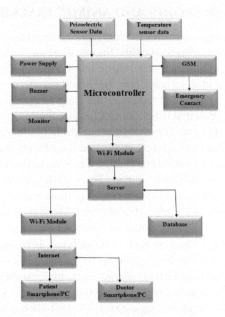

Figure 1.3 Block diagram of IoT-Based wearable system

Flask, a Python-based microweb structure, is used to create the server. Despite the word 'micro', the Flask enables extensions that can add a variety of functionalities, all of which are open source. By comparing with other basic web servers, the Flask provides simplicity and versatility. The web server runs on a Raspberry Pi "3 Model b" and uses a public IP address to connect with the database. The Raspberry Pi is a small, low-cost controller that can handle a variety of functions. CSS, JavaScript and HTML are used to create the webpages, while SQLite is used to create the database. Flask is used in collaboration with an SQLite database to store patient data for future use.

Healthcare specialists and patients can rely on the web server for validation. Specialists can view several patients' information at the same time and evaluate the overall status of an individual patient from any location which has network connectivity. Patients can now login to their account and view their real-time continuous information as well as their medical history. Later patients can send their clinical reports to the specialists for review to know about their clinical conditions and to get medical advice.

For security purposes, data from the patient's sensor is collected using a unique API. The collected data is displayed in a table with the help of Google Chart API, while a graphical representation of the data, as well as individual date–time, is available on the website. With improved number of lives saved, and because of remote checking, an expert will be able to provide therapeutic support and counselling to a larger number of people than previously.

1.4 WEARABLES IN SPORTS AND ANIMAL TRACKING

Wearables are enhancing in the mainstream, and its applications are widespread in sports, fitness and monitoring of health. Sports wearables are used in widespread applications such as monitoring pulse rate or heart rate and identifying the location. The smart phones are utilized as a hub via a cellular network which is used for observing a real-time sport. Bi-directional and long-range accessibility property of wearables, integrated with real time, doesn't require a mobile phone throughout the time period of the exercisers. These devices would help elderly people in real time to keep track of their healthy standing status and their location or site [24].

The media introduced wearable technology as a disruptive technology, which can be an ultra-player in the electronic market. The significance of this disruptive technology in wearables encompasses various types of device usage from head to toe. For example, the devices which are placed on the feet, like shoes, have motion sensors to identify gait pattern, and devices which are fixed on the head, like smart glasses or caps, have many applications; one such is identifying drowsiness and activating an anti-sleep detector to alert the driver from falling asleep [25].

In sports, fitness has gained a huge market share of consumer wearables as people are more conscious about their fitness. These wearable devices are common among most people due to the aesthetic appearance. A well-known wearable, Fitbit [26], is a digital watch which monitors the user during the time of sleep and exercise. As a lifestyle change, this wearable device has gained a major priority among the society and could recognize them to look fit. In wearable devices with regard to sports, various sensors like accelerometer, gyroscope, magnetometer, heart rate monitor, GPS and position sensors are commonly used. Accelerometers and gyroscope sensors stand ahead when compared to other sensors in the market for sports. A brief overview of the various sensors in the various brands of sports wearables is shown in Table 1.2 [27].

The accelerometer and gyroscope can give complete details regarding a sportsmen's position and can track their specific attributes. For the sports golf, the dual accelerometer and 3-axis gyroscopes can track the club speed, hip rotation and tempo ratio. In the course of the last decade, motion examination frameworks, for example video recording and PC digitization, have been utilized to quantify human motion and further develop sports execution [24]. Lot of textiles related to fitness are also available in the market. The daily activity, fitness activity, food consumption and sleep pattern are monitored with the help of the wearables in the hand. The sensors are fitted along with the wearable which helps in such remote monitoring. The data from the wearable is sent to the mobile phone which in turn is connected to the remote cloud. The data from the cloud is monitored by the caretakers, and in case of any discrepancies, it is communicated to the end-user immediately. In this way, remote monitoring of the athletes is achieved. The smart shirts designed for athletes can be used to maximize the training and performance. Inertial sensors are available to measure force and acceleration of the athlete in action. Moreover, heart rate sensors fixed along with the garments help in measuring the pulse rate of an athlete. Figure 1.4 explains the applications of a wearable in sports monitoring.

Table 1.2
Sensors Used in Various Wearable Devices

Sports Wearable	Accelerometer	Gyroscope	Magnetometer	Heart Rate Monitor	GPS
Fitbit	*		*	*	*
Fitbit	*		*	*	*
Zepp Play	*	*			*
Lumo Run	*	*			*
Optimeye	*		*	*	*
PlayerTek	*		*		*
ViperPod	*	*		*	
Adidas MiCoach	*	*			

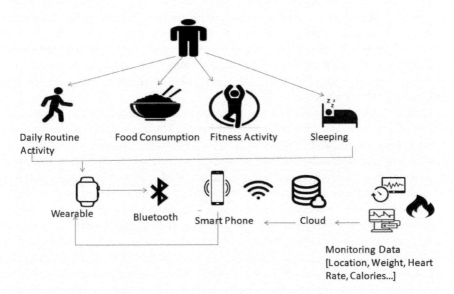

Figure 1.4 Wearable device for sports monitoring

1.4.1 RECENT INNOVATIONS IN WEARABLE DEVICES

Advances in computerized innovation are improving the creature well-being market. Applications have been created to improve the connection among veterinarians and pet proprietors. PetDialog [28] is an application that permits clients to screen practice and wholesome admission, socialization and different exercises with the assistance of an implicit schedule that conveys cautions for routine considerations like immunizations. Applications on cell phones can follow and send creature conduct and its activities to veterinarians for quicker and more precise clinical guidance. Architects at all driving organizations are creating advanced innovation to satisfy the requirements of pet proprietors, dairy ranchers and animal directors. Veterinary medical clinics were discovered ailing in online arrangement booking and online cash move frameworks, and had an unwieldy creature protection methodology, yet the new advancement of computerized frameworks is making it simpler to oversee creature well-being. Applications are likewise being intended to robotize long-standing practices in food creation. Internationally, different types of sensors are being developed for the well-being of creatures and are successful from the commercial point of view. Little advancement was also created with minimal adjustments in these devices for creatures' well-being and their infection minimization. Also, these innovative works are considered in animal health advancement [29].

1.4.2 BIOSENSORS AND THEIR APPLICATIONS

In the worldwide market, biosensors implemented for the creatures' well-being have become a developing business unit. Trend-setting innovations such as investigation of sound in various creatures, detection of sweat and saliva, procedures of picture recognition and others are used as strategies for animal cultivation. For the continuous observation of creatures' well-being, the necessity for the coordination of all accessible sensors is required to develop a productive internet checking framework. Di Gironimo et al. [30] explored different innovations for all animal beings in general. The nanosized biosensors and other analytical methods are used for spotting irresistible infections in cows.

The utilization of biosensors and wearable advancements is turning out to be progressively significant for creature well-being. These gadgets, whenever fabricated exactly and utilized effectively, can give opportune determination of illnesses in creatures, in the end diminishing monetary misfortunes. Such gadgets are especially helpful for dairy steers and poultry ranches. Rather than depending exclusively on ranchers' facilities and information, the location sensors can give solid information about the state of being of the animals. As a result of the prevalent exhibition of wearable advancements and sensors, they can make a leap forward in domesticated animals' improvement and vow to become the most significant and practicable innovation in the creature well-being market. New wearable innovations are being tweaked to address the issues of creatures, pets and domesticated animals. Items, for example prescription patches, following restraints and electronic seat improvement, are being bought at higher rates and saddled for the better childhood of livestock.

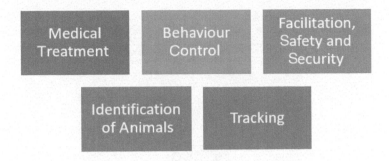

Figure 1.5   Facilities of using wearable devices

These wearable advancements are multifunctional and proficient, permitting creature proprietors to accomplish more in less time [30]. The livestock monitoring system is done by means of data acquisition. Identification and tracking of animals, medical diagnosis and behaviour monitoring can be done easily using wearable devices as shown in Figure 1.5.

1.4.3   LIVESTOCK MANAGEMENT SYSTEM

Sensors and wearable innovations can be embedded in creatures to recognize their perspiration constituents, measure internal heat level, notice conduct and development, identify pressure, examine sound, distinguish pH, forestall sickness, distinguish analytes and recognize the presence of infections and microbes. Wearable sensors help ranchers come down with sickness early, and subsequently forestall the passing of animals. Ranchers can likewise separate infected animals on schedule to forestall the spread of sickness in the entire steer groups through expectation.

One of the example of such a system is livestock management system which is shown in Figure 1.6. The biosensor module is fixed in the animal, and the data is amplified. The amplified data is communicated to the internet via a communicating module like ZigBee, Bluetooth, etc. The sensed value is transferred to the internet. The entire data management system holds the livestock values, and the analysed data is sent to the clinical support system for real-time monitoring of the data. A biosensing gadget that connects to the ears to quantify the internal heat level of creatures presently costs 100,000 US dollars for 10,000 cows. Economically accessible biosensor collars are likewise being utilized in cows for the location of oestrus period.

A creative mechanical brushing framework utilizes electronic leg groups that collaborate with sensors mounted on the creature to record information on its taking care of and draining conduct. Development and conduct of livestock can hand off data about their degree of movement and prosperity. Additionally, actual imperfections in appendages can be distinguished right on time by strange development. In enormous homesteads, depending on unaided eye perception can bring about human

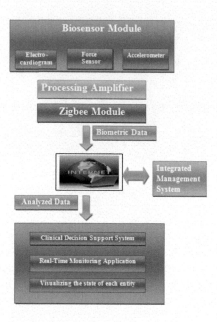

Figure 1.6   Livestock management system

mistake and a deferral in conclusion. Subsequently, better strategies for noticing ranches ought to be joined.

An innovation named MooMonitor [31] is additionally assisting ranchers with deciding the soundness of their cows through estimation of the physiological states of individual livestock. This innovation utilizes remote sensors that permit the ranchers to identify singular cow warms and well-being occasions effortlessly through information investigation. Warmth in cows and their sicknesses would thus be able to be perceived through this gadget which can help the ranchers keep their domesticated animals ideal and solid. A comparable innovation, Silent Herdsman, has been extraordinarily figured for ranchers to be utilized on livestock. Like a restraint, it's folded over the neck of every creature and directs all the exercises of cows and their practices. First it records standards of conduct, and afterwards it recognizes and records any progressions in those examples.

1.4.4   SWEAT ANALYSERS

Biosensors have been recognized as being useful in such manner; they can undoubtedly identify anti-toxin levels and caution the rancher if the anti-toxin level surpasses a most extreme reach. The biosensing innovations with the advances in the IoT worldview will advance fast, on the homestead and ongoing checking of cultivated creature sicknesses. The ongoing spread of information gathered from the homesteads through these biosensors will have esteem past the ranch also; permitting food fabricating partners' admittance to this data will be vital for the social permit issues confronting our farming area and will be a key to our proceeding with worldwide seriousness. Investigating sweat can hand off valuable data about an individual creature's well-being. Wearable perspiration analysers have not yet been made business, for the most part on account of the size imperatives of the gear. Be that as it may, minimal-expense vigorous plans have been created in research canters. Strategies for gathering sweat incorporate utilizing an electrical flow to drive a synthetic energizer into the skin iontophoresis, yet there is a requirement for techniques that gather as well as examine and screen sweat for the duration of the day or as required.

Late advancements made in sweat analysers intend to limit the size of the framework so that it is wearable and simple to deal with. Ongoing perspiration checking of sodium by expendable strips coordinated with microfluidic chips has been created; it is associated with a scaled-down remote framework to distinguish sodium levels in sweat. Checking various electrolytes all the while is more helpful; henceforth, the framework created by Gao et al. [32] passes on degrees of sodium, potassium, lactate, glucose and skin temperature all the while. Incorporated Bluetooth innovation empowers sharing and checking of the deliberate information. Biomonitoring of sweat in creatures has incredible potential for creature well-being as a result of its non-obtrusive nature. The measure of metals can likewise be recognized by sweat analysers. In the event that such an innovation is presented on ranches, changes in animal well-being can be checked in a novel design to fundamentally forestall well-being and financial misfortune.

1.5 CONCLUSIONS

Wearable sensors provide a promising solution in diverse fields. It is widely used in different fields like wellness, healthcare, industrial, gaming and military applications. In healthcare, it indicates early warnings in the detection of disease and timely intake of medicine and monitors patients with quick remedy to avoid fatality. Wearable devices can be placed anywhere on the body or inside the body. Wearable devices can be connected with the help of wireless communication technologies and interfaces. It can be concluded that remote monitoring by the wearable devices will definitely increase the number of saved lives.

2 IoT-Based Disease Prediction

Pranjal Garg and Sejal Gupta

CONTENTS

2.1 BRIEF INTRODUCTION

The pathology and its effects make the course of the disease very complex and unpredictable. Medicine is not only science but also the art of intuition and prediction on behalf of any healthcare professional. The rise of evidence-based medicine is imminent, and its dependence on data analysis cannot be exaggerated [33]. In lieu of modern advancements in computer science, the ability of machine learning (ML) to analyse data makes it a lucrative option to supplement the conventional theranostic and rehabilitation process. To intervene in healthcare management, Internet of Healthcare Things (IoHT) can provide this data through networks of many devices.

Healthcare devices can include wearables, implants, nanobots and smart pills. On the lines of wearables and implants, there could be smart bracelets, BP monitors, smart glasses, smart socks and devices that can be implanted inside a human body, like pacemakers, ventricular shunts and metallic knees. Numerous pharmaceuticals with nanobots are in different phases of development which can be consumed to diagnose or treat a particular condition [34]. These devices can transmit the patient data over a secure network from a server to cloud and fog data centres where various ML algorithms can perform various types of analytics. Another data source can be electronic health records maintained by hospitals, MedTech corporations, health insurance companies and personally by any patient.

The characteristics of any disease include aetiology, epidemiology, pathophysiology, various diagnostic modalities, intervention, prognosis and complications, if any, followed by rehabilitation. The data can provide insights and hence predict the said characteristics of disease as well as the incidence of its occurrence. For example, a blood pressure monitor will give data on the systolic and diastolic pressure of the patients using the device. Over the time, pressure data that is obtained in particular demographics with different medications can predict the prognosis of hypertension. Furthermore, the incidence can also be predicted in various age groups.

2.2   WHY IS DISEASE PREDICTION IMPORTANT?

The word disease comes from 'dis' + 'ease' which literally means 'apart from comfort'. Besides affecting health, diseases also impact us socially, economically, culturally and almost all aspects of human life. To put it simply, to live is to have a disease and hence live with the burden that comes with it. This fact makes disease prediction technology nothing less than a miracle that can derive innumerable benefits for everyone.

To establish the correspondence between disease prediction and IoHT devices, artificial intelligence (AI) techniques are necessary [35]. AI includes a computer science technique which is used to provide a mechanical and strategic solution with human-like intelligence. Several other considerations need to be taken care of before, during and after the disease prediction technique is employed, such as demographic variance, cyber security issues and consensual and appropriate use of data.

2.3   DISEASE PREDICTION STRATEGIES

IoHT envisions a scope for a new future where healthcare setups are designed to benefit the patient and provide cost-effective services. With ML and IoT as its wings, the healthcare sector will undoubtedly see immense technical progress. Smart healthcare records, disease prediction and analysis, medical diagnosis, quick, personalized prescriptions and prediction of potential pandemic outbreaks exemplify how ML will play a crucial role in medical management. In concert with IoHT, several ML algorithms are used. These include dimensionality reduction analysis like linear discriminant analysis for Parkinson's disease diagnosis, support vector machine classifiers for the identification of acute respiratory illness, monitoring of gravida with k-nearest neighbours and many more along similar lines. This chapter discusses the governance of such AI algorithms in wearable smart sensors, implants and various other applications.

ML has the power to render a drastic decrease in the use of clinical resources during lengthy researches and assay of drugs. One such common resource is animals as they are used in many stages of drug development. According to a study published in 2017 [36], the average use of animals is as much as 60–80% while characterizing the promising drug candidate. Numerous phases of trials, such as identifying possible medicines, concept testing and lead identification, require resources in terms of life, time and money. The assay of drugs can be made more accurate and efficient using ML algorithms and neural networks. This can be used effectively as strategized data points can be generated, and their effects can be studied based on analysis and prediction models through case studies. The use of such varied strategies and models could minimize the in vivo trials and replicate the behaviour of research subjects in a machine-friendly environment.

Disease prediction can happen at the following levels: individual, institutional, district, state, national and international. Segregating and analysing data at various levels can help identify aetiology and contain the infection within that region. IoT is known among technologists for producing a large volume of data. IoT with ML and deep learning can prove tremendously progressive as more the data, more accessible the training and smoother the prediction. Thus, the application of IoT integrated with ML models in the prediction of the prognosis of common diseases and the future disease outbreaks will render increased efficacy of new plausible treatments.

2.4 ENVIRONMENT: HEALTHCARE SETUPS, SMART DEVICES AND SOURCE OF DATA

In the following subsections, the overall environment for setting up of IoHT-like healthcare setups, smart devices that can be involved in the IoHT and source of data for analysis purpose is discussed.

2.4.1 HEALTHCARE SETUPS

Healthcare services are disseminated in a wide array of settings including emergency rooms, outpatient departments, inpatient units, hospices, rehabilitation centres, surgical clinics, home-based services, etc. Moreover, diagnostic laboratories such as pathology-based labs, microbiology-based labs, imaging labs like X-rays, MRI or CT or PET-based scanning facilities, EEG labs, ECG labs and others on similar lines provide support to healthcare professionals in making the correct diagnosis.

The healthcare facilities can also be divided into five major categories: primary healthcare centres (PHCs), secondary healthcare centres (SHCs), tertiary healthcare centres (THCs), quarternary healthcare centres (QHCs) and point of care (POC) services. It is necessary to identify such levels to obtain data categorically, do a market evaluation and eventually roll out efficient IoHT devices for use in disease prediction. For example, it is often difficult to target PHCs as they cater to the significantly mild form of diseases like the common cold, mild flu and allergies, where IoHT has

Table 2.1
Devices Used to Predict Diseases

Medical Devices	Pathologies
Heart rate monitors	Atrial fibrillation, atrial flutter and conduction blocks
Blood Pressure Monitors	Hypertension, hypotension and pheochromocytoma
Smart Shoes	Propulsive gait and spastic gait
Smart headsets	Otitis externa and progressive hearing impairment
Smart Ventriculoperitoneal Shunts	Hydrocephalus and slit ventricular syndrome
Cochlear Implants	Hearing impairments
Knee Replacement Implants	Surgical site infections and allergies
Pacemaker	Long QT syndrome
Dental implants	Gum infections, oral infections and systemic infections

negligible applicability. Though PHC can play an indispensable role in promulgating awareness regarding IoT devices, intuitively, they cannot attract the attention of a large populace [37]. On the other hand, POC and THC can provide data to lay a true cornerstone to revolutionize disease prediction [38].

2.4.2   COMMON HEALTHCARE-ASSOCIATED WEARABLES AND IMPLANTS

The data collected from almost all IoHT wearables and implants can be used for disease prediction. Table 2.1 illustrates some of these devices and diseases that can be used for the same. However, it is noteworthy that these devices will require additional data to indicate any characteristic of the disease.

2.4.3   IMPORTANT DATA TYPES FOR IoHT

Healthcare produces data from numerous sources like individuals, medical service providers, health insurance companies and national health agencies like the Centre for Disease Control and Prevention. Individuals with implants and wearables can provide healthcare data to the cloud. Similarly, medical service providers like diagnostic laboratories with high-tech machines like automated haematology analysers, health insurance companies with data on patient financials and associated medical history, and national agencies with millions of data points on population medical records, vaccination status and disease outbreaks are all different sources of data.

The data provided by healthcare providers can be of different types. The type of ML algorithm and the pre=processing steps that need to be employed in these data types will depend on the data type. Figure 2.1 illustrates some of the standard algorithms that are witnessed in healthcare settings. The IoT device used to collect the data and send it to the cloud will also rely on the collected data. Only with a combination of all these data types, an accurate disease prediction can be made. For example, the myocardial infarction needs both signal data (ECG) and blood reports (troponin protein) and patient medical history to make accurate predictions and the type of medical care needed.

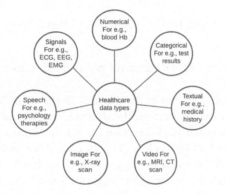

Figure 2.1 IoHT: Healthcare data types prominently used in disease prediction and analysis

2.4.4 SOURCE OF DATA TYPES PRODUCED IN HEALTHCARE SETTINGS

The type of data used in IoHT can be from three different sources as shown in Figure 2.2.

When getting data from **passive sources**, the sensor is not actively sending signals over the cloud. It needs to be activated when the user intends to transmit data. For example, the usage of manual glucometers in POC settings that detect blood sugar levels can be turned on once the required blood glucose levels are collected. From **active sources**, the sensors transmit data in real time with the use of sophisticated IoT communication technologies. The fear of data loss is minimal in active sources, as the data is consumed instantly. For example, heart rate monitors worn by runners can communicate heart rate to the cloud as the user continues wearing the device. These **dynamic sources** not only transmit data in real time but also allow the base station to converse with the source and modify the data to meet the demands of the base station. It is also possible to fibrillate cardiac arrest patients using implanted

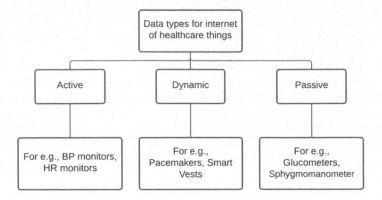

Figure 2.2   Source of data for the application of IoHT devices.

devices or smart vests; however, extensive pre-clinical studies are required to make a marketable product.

To predict the characteristics of the disease, all three kinds of data types can be used. From a healthcare perspective, the dynamic sources provide theranostic capabilities, which, if administered according to the standards of medical ethics, will form the upper berth of all types of IoT capabilities. After that, both active and passive sources can equally mitigate the risk of disease outbreaks and prevent emergencies. For example, diabetes is one of the significant troublemakers for public health professionals. The digital glucometers help recognize pre-diabetic patients, and the resources can be released by public health agencies accordingly. Similarly, the effectiveness of drugs that are administered for diabetes can also be assessed, giving a boost to evidence-based medicine.

2.5   CHARACTERISTICS OF A DISEASE

Several parameters like aetiology, epidemiology, pathophysiology, diagnostic modalities, intervention, prognosis, complications and rehabilitation define a disease. The prediction of a disease is based on the conjecture of these parameters. Hence, to avail the benefits of IoHT devices for disease prediction, it is vital to know about the data types created in the healthcare system and the disease parameters to which that data refers.

Aetiology defines the causation of disease and lays out the fundamentals to describe its origin [39]. For example, infectious diseases like the common cold are caused by rhinoviruses, tuberculosis by Mycobacterium and diptheria by Corynebacterium. Similarly, other conditions might have some causative microorganism or other complex aetiologies. For instance, sensors enabled with the Internet of Bio-Nano Things that detect the quorum sensing communication between infectious agents are used to deduce the infection even before the symptoms arise in the infected patient [40]. IoT-Based prediction of any disease's aetiology helps pre-clinical scientists define the cause of a disease with unknown aetiology. Identifying the correlation of the disease with its probable causes is the first step in treating a disease. The data for the same can be collected by high-risk patients wearing smart IoT devices.

Epidemiology is a branch of medical science dealing with several diseased individuals in a particular location, time or demographic. It tells public health professionals about the changing number of diseased individuals and how it impacts the area's economy [41]. The biggest challenge in conducting epidemiological studies is collecting accurate data from all the possible sources. Importantly, epidemiology is a continuously changing parameter that requires constant monitoring. IoT devices can enhance our ability to evaluate this change by several manifolds. It is also possible to predict any epidemiological variable of unknown diseases if we have information about other conditions with similar pathologies. Noteworthily, epidemiological studies might also be helpful in conducting market research for IoHT devices.

The loci of convergence of pathology of any disease and associated physiology refer to *pathophysiology*. It studies the aberration that affects the physiology of disease. It lays down the processes that allow biomedical scientists to identify novel therapeutic techniques. Unlike other parameters, the pathophysiology is a complex blend of interconnected biological processes that requires systemic data at the cellular level besides macroscopic data points. The data extraction with smart wearables at the macroscopic level and IoT-enabled implants can play a significant role in collecting data to identify pathophysiologies of complex diseases [42]. For example, a real-time healthcare monitoring Bio-IoT (RTBioT) is a new pre-clinical platform that quantifies chromophores in human tissues using near-infrared spectroscopy. This platform can be used for detecting the pathophysiology of melanomas, anemia or porphyria [43]. Internet of Bio-Nano Things, which performs at the bio-cyber interface, can be another suitable design for discovering complex pathophysiology.

Various *diagnostic* modalities like clinical examination, pathological and microbiological examinations and imaging techniques are employed by physicians to identify the disease. IoHT devices in lieu of existing diagnostic procedures can be utilized to prepare a differential diagnosis and accurately predict diseases. As IoT allows continuous monitoring of symptoms, it also enables a rapid, cost-efficient and accurate diagnostic. For example, classification algorithms have been used to predict strokes among high-risk stroke patients on the data collected from IoT sensors designed to monitor blood pressure [44].

Intervention is any procedure or action undertaken by healthcare professionals to alter the course of any illness to provide relief to the patients. Intervention can be in the form of drugs, non-pharmacological therapies and surgery. IoT can play a significant role in predicting the best treatment which can be offered to the patients. Continuous monitoring of symptoms can evaluate the efficacy of therapy. One such program is Mental Health IoT, which allows confidential behavioural therapy for patients with depression and anxiety [45]. This can provide swift care to high suicide-risk patients. Due to substantial variable pharmacogenomics, side effects can be commonly seen among different forms of therapy. The continuous monitoring of the efficacy of a specific treatment empowers the implementation of personalized medicine, wherein healthcare delivery is tailored for individual needs with minimal side effects.

Prognosis is the expected course of a medical condition that is often based on the combination of medical facts, medical data and the physician's intuition. It predicts the prospect of developing a condition in an individual and speculates the survivability of a patient after being diagnosed with a fatal disease. Coherent prediction of medical prognostics allows the patient and physician to decide on the therapeutic strategy suitable for the patient or decide on hospice care in case of the untreatable fatal disease [46]. For example, prognosis in the palliative care study (PiPS) model is a new strategy that can predict the median survival; however, targeted clinical studies are required with IoT-enabled sensors for complete implementation [47]. When prognostic analysis fails to predict the course of the disease, complications arise that become challenging to manage. The use of glucose sensors to prevent the case of diabetic retinopathy is an instance where IoHT can be specifically used to predict and avoid the complication of diabetes mellitus.

Rehabilitation reduces disability and allows patients to regain optimal functioning following an illness, injury or any debilitating medical condition. Rehabilitation requirements vary from patient to patient and from a medical condition to another. An example of IoT-Based prediction of rehabilitation needs can be sports. A strategy has been developed where the wearable sensor–based fuzzy decision-making (FDM) model seamlessly monitors a sportsperson's physical activity, allowing rehabilitation centres to monitor physical activity and predict the rehabilitation requirements [48].

2.5.1 PREDICTING PANDEMICS, EPIDEMICS, ENDEMICS AND OUTBREAKS

Pandemics, epidemics and endemics suggest the outbreak of a disease in a particular area at a particular time with different levels of prevalence [49]. Timely and accurate identification and prediction of such outbreaks can prevent thousands or even millions of people from probable fatal or disabling diseases. Many times, traditional methods fail to tackle the menace of widespread outbreaks due to a lack of temporal data from different demographics. For example, in the case of communicable diseases like dengue fever, influenza A, yellow fever and COVID-19, public health officials resort to quarantine and largely untested immunizations. Due to lack of evidence, these strategies intuitively only provide substandard relief to the affected individuals [50]. The IoHT network provides a robust framework to materialize the promise of prevention of such pandemics or at the very least prepare for the upcoming outbreak incidences. For example, a flu prediction machine for the prediction of the influenza pandemic has been proposed [51]. It gains from BSN-Care, a body sensor network based on IoHT.

2.6 DETAILED LITERATURE REVIEW

The following subsection provides an insight into the IoT-Based sensors and methodologies used in the prediction and analysis of a disease. It also provides a comprehensive overview of the existing IoHT applications.

2.6.1 ALZHEIMER'S DISEASE

The first review is about the prediction of Alzheimer's in the geriatric population. It is estimated that nearly 44 million people worldwide live with Alzheimer's disease or some form of dementia [52]. This disease is on an increasing trend, and with optimal analytics tools to predict the course of Alzheimer's in high-risk people, a better plan of action to tackle the threat can be developed. Today, medications and effective support strategies are the only ways to reduce and control the symptomatic conditions. The peril of Alzheimer's is developed by the pounding risk of heart disease and high blood pressure in the patients. Researchers worldwide are trying to come up with the solutions such as prediction of Alzheimer's disease in accordance with the analysis of daily activities of the patients to graph out statistics that can help prognosticate luring dangers of Alzheimer's or dementia.

The discussion by Chong et al. [53] uses projections of three types of variables to curate a behavioural analysis model based on sensors collecting data of 20 elderly living in flats alone for over six months. The first variable evaluates the activity level of a person. Empirical research revealed that high variance in graphs leads to a positive case. The second variable in this study signifies an individual's sleep patterns. If the research subject does not have a regular sleep pattern and has a spike in activity levels during the night than during the day, then the person may be indicative of Alzheimer's symptoms. The third variable which was taken into consideration in this research was the amount of repetition in behaviour. Study on Alzheimer's patients shows immense similarity in their work. Their recapitulations in both verbal and non-verbal actions are empirically studied. Thus the third variable is calculated based on their similarity in their various activities.

Visual analytics is performed over IoT data by extraction, transformation and loading (ETL). The sensors detect the movements of the subjects within the parameters of the house. Video analysis of their actions and behaviours is carried out to fill the table of the three variables. Each registered behaviour represented by time, location and action was recorded with a unique id. Using graphical and prediction analysis tools, the records were analysed, and the potential risk of Alzheimer's was detected. The stages of the design use data warehouse and analysis tools such as MS SQL Studio (data cleaning and ETL), Tableau (data visualization) and heatmaps from the Tableau (prediction analysis). By constantly mapping the patients' activities, the prediction model categorizes them into three groups of Alzheimer's risk: abnormal, potential and normal. For Alzheimer's prediction, a color matrix for all the three variables and a risk rating matrix for each patient are drawn out. A profile of these patients is chartered by applying levels of problem detection.

The tests infer that the second variable of sleep patterns turns out ineffective due to numerous reasons. The solution design thus effectively takes up the first and the third variables and states them as the constituting factors leading to the solutions.

2.6.2 PANDEMIC PREDICTION USING BIG DATA ANALYTICS

This review is about pandemic prediction with the integrated use of IoT and big data analytics . The recent COVID-19 pandemic has shaped the research industry in finding meaning in every new detail related to patients. This review supports discussions in various works done by authors in [54–57]. The prediction and analysis of the next sensitive outbreak and the prevention and the rich critical role of medics in preparedness are discussed. This discussion reviews extensive neural networks, early research data of patients of COVID-19 and humongous structured data of patients with varied attributes and symptoms. The works mentioned above examine the substantial effect of data analysis, prediction and aetiology of the disease.

The methodologies and environment put into use are IoT sensors. The IoT-Based framework leverages the use of cloud and fog computing systems to deliver and store data. The data from these sensors is then mined for extensive data analysis using ensemble ML techniques, AI algorithms and neural networks. Numerous heuristic methods have also been put to use to examine potential threats. The empirical research performed on wearable IoHT devices for comprehensive healthcare observation has proven [36] to be a crucial part of predicting pandemics.

A framework has been prepared for pandemic prediction by breaking down the analysis into some simplified modules; descriptive, diagnostic, predictive and prescriptive analysis [54]. The data collected from the sensors and monitoring devices is aggregated and then passed through respective analysis modules. The illustrative analysis modules perform attribute selection and extraction before visualizing the data. This is followed by diagnostic analysis, which is a crucial stage as the most filtered data is passed through it before prediction analysis. In healthcare, this step helps in analysing the data to diagnose symptoms and make other correlations using attributes extracted in the first step. The diagnostic analysis of data is carried out using data mining and data discovery. This interpreted data is evaluated through a trained model and a learned model to estimate the likelihood of an outbreak. The use of random forest and decision tree algorithms can help formulate the spread rate of disease.

The diagnosed data set is divided into training and testing data sets. The training module passes through deep learning networks and ML models, whereas the test set passes through a learning module. The deep learning modules include the backpropagation and feed-forward neural network. The evaluation parameters are also analysed to verify and predict the results, facilitating better prescriptive analysis. Using these modules, a pandemic can be predicted and detected by comparing the effects of patients through neural networks. A graph of positive and negative tests is drawn out to infer the possibility of a pandemic.

The IoT sensors produce a lot of data from various sources. Data of the patients can be effectively proctored to detect any new symptoms, prediction, prescription and analysis. Such analyses are significant in understanding the naive and any upcoming disease by visualizing the analysed data graphically.

2.6.3 SYMPTOM ANALYSIS AND DISEASE PREDICTION

The following review is based on IoT-Based wearable sensors for symptom analysis and disease prediction. Analysis of big data has been proven to be of significance as a prediction of market trends and meaningful patterns from unstructured data have all become accessible and advantageous. Consequential insights such as disease prediction and symptom analysis have rendered life-changing directions to the healthcare sector. A large volume of data is collected via numerous IoT sensors installed at different places, starting from smartphones to offices and hospitals, and even the human body. These sensors measure human states, such as monitoring heart rate, physical activity trackers, etc., and can amount to millions of data points every minute. The data is extensively surveyed to direct its usage in diagnosing chronic ailments, predicting pandemics and analysing symptoms. Upon research and consent, wearable sensors can produce data to predict if a person is healthy or not and verify their nutritional intake. Numerous such as aptasensors are also helpful in monitoring sleep cycles, heart rate, blood pressure and food intake; all these can help in symptom analysis. The first discussion in this subsection can also be further improvized and advanced manifolds with monitoring wearables for human vitals. Since the wearables could be non-invasive and voluntarily controllable by the patients, they are the more accepted and cost-effective techniques to detect and prevent illness.

IoT wearables produce real-time data in big data storage centres. Once this data is pre-processed, it is sent to analyse and classify information using AI training models. Muthu et al. [58] used a Generalized Approximate Reasoning-based Intelligence Control (GARIC) implemented with regression rules to perform intelligent symptom analysis. ML regressors and classifiers are self-learning, and the power of performing correlation among symptoms is highly significant. This paper explicitly used a Boltzmann belief neural network to train the data. Disease prediction is then performed via a regularization genome-wide association study (GWAS). These neural nets render the prediction model definitive and trustworthy. Subsequently, if a patient is diagnosed, they receive digital updates and treatment methodologies by connecting to hospitals.

The security and network infrastructure of the data models should be reliant and secure. To achieve an intelligent connection between the heterogeneous devices, Istepanian et al. [59] suggested to use new communication routes for through an advanced IP-based networking architecture. Numerous transport protocols implement cryptographic algorithms to prevent insecure breaches and data leaks. Apart from a safe and riveted architecture, dynamic segmentation of prediction models also helped in a thorough analysis of the disease.

2.6.4   SECURITY-RELATED THREATS

The following review is based on security-related threats in IoHT and their impact on the healthcare sector. IoHT has prominently proved to perform an essential role in unifying the medical infrastructure and IoT. It has revolutionized the industry by applying health proctoring, handling emergency conditions, symptom analysis, disease prediction and even predicting pandemic outbreaks. With benefits come disadvantages. The high volume of data under investigation might be very private information of the patients. Digitalization is susceptible to numerous security threats and implicates the area of study, for example the healthcare sector or financial markets.

Table 2.2
Analysis of Security Breaches in IoHT

Type of Attack	Requirements	Solution
Denial of Service Attack	Early intrusion detection	Authentication and authorization should be the prime focus, but in the case of DDoS or DoS, system services should be disabled to prevent leaks.
Location-Based Attack (Fingerprint and Timing-Based Snooping (FATS))	Secured firewalls and installation of honeypots	The misled transmission of information can be controlled by installation of firewalls and antivirus protection.
Sensor Attack	Secured network protocol	Authentication mechanisms to secure network and communication lines.
Replay Attack	Secure Authorization	To secure the data from ill monitoring, the false packets could be dropped by measuring their false timestamps.

Being such a crucial sector, data in healthcare is private and personal, henceforth, vulnerable to high risk. Avinashiappan et al. [60] discussed data breaches, leaks and malwares that disrupt the integrity of the data. Since hospitals, data centres and even insurance ventures would be interconnected with IoT sensors, the data leaks will pound a potential threat on a large quarter of society. These threats include hampering both the network and transport protocol.

Rathee et al. [61] prove that blockchain provisions a secure healthcare management system by generating the hash of each data to provide a series of certain records only accessible on the patient's networks. It provides a hybrid and safe framework for processing multimedia. Blockchain accounts for the non-repudiation, accessibility and traceability of records. Table 2.2 shows a brief representation on the types of attack and generic solutions.

2.7 FUTURE DIRECTIONS

There is a lot of scope for IoHT in future. A few of the possible future directions in this area are summarized in Table 2.3.

Table 2.3
Applications of IoHT and Future Directions

Applications	Future directions
Diagnostics	Integration of all monitoring systems, including electronic health records, health insurance records, smart wearables and pharmacy records to perform an accurate diagnosis.
Prognostic evaluation	Development of well-trained and efficient AI algorithms to supplement the physician's experience.
Intervention Prediction	Intervention warrants both responsibility and accountability on behalf of all the stakeholders involved in providing medical advice. Intervention tends to have serious adverse effects. This requires significant collaboration efforts between not only the institutional-level healthcare workers and IoT engineers but also between different departments of policymakers.
Personalized Care	Personalized care is seen with hostility among many patients, and they often portray serious concerns over privacy issues, data theft, cyber security and among others. As a result, this demands effort towards confidence building, the development of customized cryptography algorithms or the introduction of hardware-based microelectronics to protect data.
Pathophysiology prediction	The work at the microscopic level projects the major driving force in determining pathophysiology. None of the IoBNT sensors have yet received FDA clearance. Therefore, it is still at a very nascent stage where the gap in basic science is very evident.

2.8 CONCLUSIONS

The use of IoT-enabled sensors for disease prediction seems no less than a miracle. It is a cause of major excitement among both the medical fraternity and IoT engineers. The gap between the proposed structures and the current practicalities threatens the execution of IoHT-driven disease prediction. The majority of this gap is formed by a lack of IoT-Based pre-clinical studies and hence the clinical trials. Newer and more advanced paradigms of ML algorithms are also required to enhance the prediction capabilities as the medical application requires highly accurate prediction techniques. Modern technologies like AI and IoT uncover a seemingly phenomenal ability that empowers healthcare workers to benefit from millions of data points about the medical condition of their patients. The data collected is then subject to analysis by AI techniques like ML and deep learning. In this chapter, first the data types usually available in healthcare settings and the disease parameters that these data types describe are discussed. Next, commonly used wearables and implants that can be associated with the prediction of disease are explored. Then the strategies employed to make accurate predictions of disease and a few examples where such methods have already been deployed are discussed. A combination of several data types with millions of data points from a single individual is required to predict disease. As a result, the collaboration of multiple data centres, rehabilitation centres, pharmacies, etc., is needed to implement the strategies discussed in this chapter.

3 An Introduction to IoT-Based Posture Detection and Underlying Sensor Technology

Jahnvi Gupta, Nitin Gupta, Mukesh Kumar and Ritwik Duggal

CONTENTS

3.1 INTRODUCTION

Stanford Health News defines 'posture' as the way your muscles and skeleton hold the body erect. It can also be defined as the position in which a person holds their

DOI: 10.1201/9781003239895-3

body upright against gravity when standing, sitting, walking or performing any activity. Maintaining a good posture is vital to the overall health of all human beings. Negligence towards maintaining a good posture can cause many life-threatening conditions such as shoulder and back pains, reduced lung function, gastrointestinal pains, scoliosis, postural syndrome, etc. Prolonged bad posture has a very severe negative impact on any person's day-to-day or work life.

People generally do not seek medication until an acute pain is felt. The treatment then may range from some rest and physiotherapy to even surgery depending on the severity of the issue. Thus, large amount of money is spent on such treatments which could have avoided in the first place if proper precautions had been taken. Therefore, posture and posture analysis are important issues. Posture analysis, as the name describes, is a process of examining the posture of a person, and based on the posture, it can be concluded if a person is healthy or unhealthy.

In posture detection, the posture of a person is classified as a good or a bad, based on his current activity. Apart from this, another way to analyse the health of a person by his/her posture is posture recognition, where the activity patterns (sitting, standing and lying) can be analysed to judge the overall health of a person. Activity monitoring through posture recognition or detection also forms an integral part of ambient-assisted living systems for the elderly and can be used for fall detection.

3.2   TYPES OF POSTURE DETECTION TECHNIQUES

After the overview of posture analysis, an overview of different types of methods available for posture detection is presented in this section. The two broad approaches available presently for detecting the posture of a person are as follows:

1. **Invasive Methods:** Invasive methods are those which require the use of instruments inside or on the body of the subject, i.e. the sensors may be implanted within the body or attached to the surface of the body for posture detection. For posture detection, wearables are more commonly used [62]. Wearables that are very popular include iwatches, fitness bands, etc., which are used by people to monitor day-to-day health parameters such as blood pressure, heart rate, etc.

2. **Non-invasive Methods:** Non-invasive methods are those which do not require the use of any wearable sensors or device to detect postures, for example using cameras to collect information about the posture of a person. This will then rely on the use of computer vision techniques to detect and classify postures. First of all the principal body parts which are the extremities of the body such as head, feet and hands are detected. Based on these detections, then the secondary body parts are searched, i.e. shoulders, elbows and knees.

3.2.1   INVASIVE VS. NON-INVASIVE

The advantage of the non-invasive methods is that these provide lesser hindrance to the user. Moreover, these methods give higher accuracy than the non-invasive methods and are less likely to be affected by external environmental conditions. These can also be used for a variety of activities and are not limited to a few. Thus invasive methods are more suitable for real-time applications than non-invasive methods. Further, invasive methods may hinder the activities of a person in day-to-day scenario (depending on the size and position of the sensor), and working of the systems is based highly on a subject's willingness to wear the sensors.

On the other hand, non-invasive methods are prone to lesser accuracy than the invasive methods. The non-invasive methods (cameras) may also be affected by the external environmental conditions like the lighting of a room [63], the angle at which a subject is facing the detector or any other obstructions in the room. Apart from this, large computational requirements are required to handle the images, often rendering the solution unsustainable for real-time applications. Thus depending on the application, invasive or non-invasive methods can be used accordingly.

3.3 SENSOR-BASED METHODS FOR POSTURE DETECTION

Generally, there are two main methods of using sensors for posture detection:

1. **Calculation of the pressure distribution over various weight dividing surfaces:** This is a non-invasive approach in which sensors are placed on the sitting/lying surface and not on the body of the subject itself.

2. **Calculation of the angular difference between current posture and a predetermined good posture:** This is a non-invasive approach in which sensors are placed on the body of the subjects.

For the first (pressure-based) approach as described in [64], strength and ultrasonic sensors are used. The authors proposed an approach for analysing the posture in only sitting position. First of all, a comfortable and height-appropriate chair according to the subject is selected, such that they maintain a good posture for data collection. The chair selection is described as an important step such that the subjects reach their natural state where the spine position and the space between the vertebrae do not differ and the waist and back muscles stay relaxed. Generally, the *Arduino* platform is used for the implementation of the system not only because it is a powerful embedded system but also very versatile in nature.

Once the data are collected, they are fed to a machine learning (ML) algorithm like K-nearest neighbour algorithm (KNN). Because the number of features is very large, another algorithm principal component analysis (PCA) may also be used for dimensionality reduction. Figure 3.1 shows the stages for data collection and analysis.

This approach is limited to sitting posture where sensors can be installed inside the chair to acquire data. This can be beneficial for the scenario where people or students work for a long time at desk without causing any hindrance. It can also be used for patients on the wheelchair. The limitation of this method is that it cannot help in correcting the posture or detection throughout.

In the second approach, wearable sensors like accelerometer are used to measure the acceleration along x, y and z axis at the point where it is placed on the body [65].

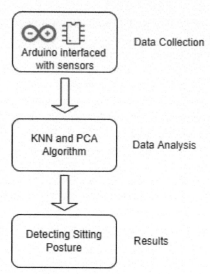

Figure 3.1   Data collection and analysis

Along with it, gyroscope may also be used to measure angular velocity along x, y and z direction. These values can then be transmitted to a computing model through wires or wireless medium (through WiFi or Bluetooth) for further processing and classification [66].

Generally, a belt is designed which consists of a sensor network comprising of an accelerometer and gyroscope: accelerometer for measuring the tilt of the body and gyroscope for measuring the movement of the body. Then Bluetooth module is used for connecting the belt containing these sensors to the mobile application designed to display these readings. This application then alerts the user if he/she is exhibiting a good or a bad posture.

Further, serial port programming has been done in [65] to get the particular output on the *Arduino*. The programming in the *Arduino* has been done for different gestures and positions of the body that a person undergoes in routine life. Figure 3.2 depicts the basic design of a posture belt.

A very similar approach like the posture belt described in [65] has been used in [67]. The authors describe the design and development of a wearable Smart Rehabilitation Garment (SRG) for posture detection and analysis. This sensor-based garment is also connected to a mobile application via Bluetooth and alerts the user by buzzing an alarm when the user is exhibiting a bad posture.

In another wearable sensor-based approach by Lim et al. [68], two accelerometers are placed on different parts of a person's spine. Apart from accelerometer, two other sensors that are also used in this approach are goniometer and electrogoniometer. A goniometer is a device that is used by a doctor or physical therapy to measure the range of motion (ROM) around a joint in the body. The goniometer is a manual device and cannot store the data, and thus the electrogoniometer was invented. This

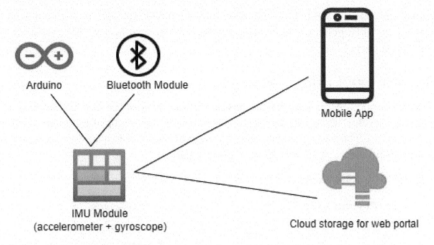

Figure 3.2   Schematic structure of posture belt [65]

device shows a high precision by $\pm 0.1^0$ for all different ROM angles and can evaluate six types of movement directions and five different angles for a given movement direction. The authors mentioned that gyroscope would help in providing more information but was not used such that system does not become more bulky and also power is not highly drained.

The other two sensors, goniometer and electrogoniometer, help in the calculation of angle, leading to the determination of posture. This design is simple, effective and wearable, but is only implemented on sitting positions. After interfacing the accelerometer with *Arduino*, authors performed three experiments on the subject. **Experiment I**: Calibration test to compare the accelerometer with goniometer, **Experiment II**: Measurement performance test to compare the accelerometer angle with electrogoniometer and **Experiment III**: Real-time system analysis.

In a novel solution presented in [69] and [70], a custom-designed wireless body area sensor network (WBASN), called WiMoCA, has been used. WiMoCA sensing node is designed to be a wearable sensor and is a low-power module providing fast update of each component. It also gives the complete implementation of a distributed posture recognition application.

One very innovative, application-specific way for posture detection where the computer users are warned when they lean too close to the computer is the 'Postuino' [71]. Here the sensors are placed next to the computer screen and not on the body of the user. This innovative approach helps the user to keep a safe distance from the electronic screen, but does not detect the overall posture as a healthy or unhealthy one.

3.4   SENSOR TECHNOLOGY FOR POSTURE DETECTION

Next, in order to understand the working of the sensors, the underlying technology is required to be understood. This section will elaborate the underlying technology for various sensors and will help in the selection of appropriate sensors for posture detection. Currently, generally micro electro-mechanical systems (MEMS) technology is used in sensors [72].

3.4.1 INTRODUCTION TO MEMS

MEMS is a microtechnology, as the physical dimension range is less than one micrometre, therefore even smaller in comparison with the width of a human hair (75 micrometre). Electro-mechanical refers to the fact that it consists of the actuator in the chip itself. Broadly, it consists of two main parts:

1. **Microsensing element**: This part accepts the input signal.

2. **Transduction Unit**: This part gets the power supply as well as manages the output.

Accelerometer and gyroscope, are examples of MEMS technology. Figure 3.3 depicts a simple representation of MEMS.

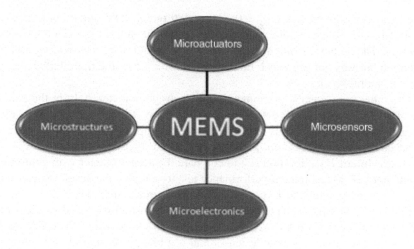

Figure 3.3   A representation of MEMS

3.4.2 ACCELEROMETER

Next, in this subsection, accelerometer is discussed in detail. An accelerometer is a device that is used to measure acceleration forces in all the 3-axis, i.e. X-axis, Y-axis and Z-axis. The force may be static, such as in the case of gravity, but mostly the dynamic forces are used such that vibrations/movement can be sensed. Figure 3.4 shows the composition of an accelerometer.

This work can be seen in everyday items such as smartphones as a luxury, or in a car's mechanism of opening the airbags. Basically, the data are taken and decided what is to be done, for which signal processing chip connected to the accelerometer

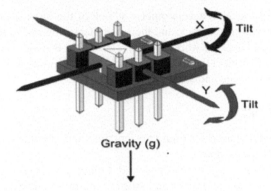

Figure 3.4 Representation of an accelerometer

is used usually. In order to achieve this, piezoresistive materials are used, which are basically materials that exhibit a change in resistance as a result of an applied strain and generally termed as strain gauges. Further, Gauge factor is the relative change in the resistance per unit strain [73].

There are two modes of resistance change; when strain is applied, the device is deformed.

1. Physical change in dimensions.

2. Resistivity, which is a function of strain.

Physical change contributes to the gauge factor majorly, in case of metal strain gauge. Change in resistivity of the material dominantly contributes to the gauge factor in case of piezoresistive strain gauge, which are semiconductor-based strain gauges. Figure 3.5 shows the variation of stress with respect to change in gauge.

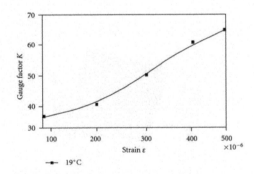

Figure 3.5 Graph of stress vs. gauge

These methods make an accelerometer as one of the most widely used sensors. They also give very high accuracy, and their manufacturing and efficient use is made possible by MEMS. Once the working of accelerometer is understood, it can be used in the correct way to collect the required data. While collecting data for postures, the data should be as accurate and sensitive as possible.

3.4.3   GYROSCOPE

It is basically, a device used for finding orientation and angular velocity. Figure 3.6 shows a digram of gyroscope.

Initially, vibrating ring gyroscopes and tuning fork gyroscopes were used. MEMS gyroscopes soon took over and still are the most widely produced. One of the most widely used MEMS gyroscopes is the Piezoelectric Plate Gyroscope which uses a lead zirconate titanate (PZT) plate as its base. At microlevels, an entire plate is made of piezoelectric material. It requires a much smaller drive voltage to create readable outputs, in comparison with its predecessors. Generally a piezoelectric plate has a length and width much more than its depth. This plate has electrical leads connected to all six sides and is placed on top of a thin membrane of a cavity in a silicon wafer. The cavity allows more freedom for the PZT to vibrate and deform. The leads provide the driving voltage and measure the output.

The sheet does not vibrate like a plate or fork. An AC driving voltage is applied vertically across the plate and also the thickness of the plate vibrates, which also oscillates with time and hence creates vibration. When the vibrating plate is rotated about an axis perpendicular to the drive voltage, a voltage is produced in the third perpendicular direction. This output voltage is proportional to the angular velocity.

This subsection helped to understand the importance of placing gyroscope at the right position and at the right orientation. MEMS technology provides very high sensitivity, and thus high precision can be acquired. Further, *vibrating-ring gyroscope* is another popular gyroscope and mainly used in cars. It can also be used according to the requirement.

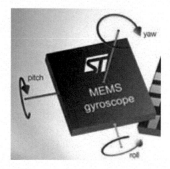

Figure 3.6   An example of a gyroscope

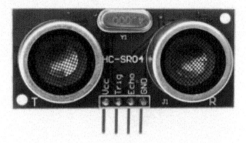

Figure 3.7   Ultrasonic Distance Sensor Module (HC SR04)

3.4.4   ULTRASONIC SENSOR

An ultrasonic sensor is one of the most commonly sensor used to measure the distance. Figure 3.7 shows an ultrasonic distance sensor module, and Figure 3.8 shows the working of the ultrasonic sensors.

It has basically two parts, the transmitter (left side in the Figure 3.7) and the receiver (right side in the Figure 3.7). The transmitter is the source of the ultrasonic waves. These waves are at much higher frequency for the humans to hear. When these waves hit an object, they are reflected back. When the receiver detects these waves after reflection, the distance can be computed by the time it takes for the waves to return using Equation (3.1),

$$\text{Distance} = \left(\frac{1}{2} \times \text{Time} \right) \times \text{Speed of light}. \tag{3.1}$$

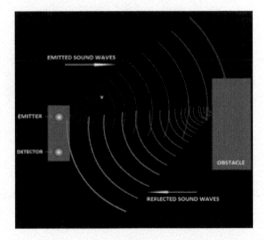

Figure 3.8   An image showing the working of the ultrasonic sensor

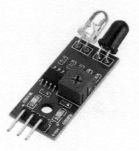

Figure 3.9   A real-life IR proximity sensor

This is used while measuring the distance of different points, like to measure the distance of the spine from different parts of the chair, when the person is sitting on it.

3.4.5   IR DISTANCE SENSOR

IR distance sensor is one of the most common sensors used for object detection. The key difference between IR distance sensor and ultrasonic sensor is that mostly IR sensor is used just to detect the object and not to measure the distance. Ultrasonic sensor offers more range, as well as accuracy, but the IR sensor has its own advantages such as low cost. Figure 3.9 shows an IR sensor, and Figure 3.10 depicts the working of an IR sensor.

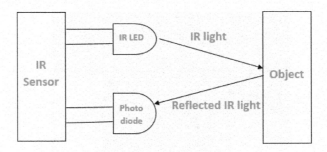

Figure 3.10   A schematic diagram showing how an IR sensor works

In the infrared spectrum, all the objects radiate some form of thermal radiation. An infrared sensor can detect these radiations where the emitter is simply an IR LED and the detector is simply an IR photodiode. A photodiode is sensitive to IR light of the same wavelength which is emitted by the IR LED. As the IR light falls on the photodiode, the resistances and the output voltages change in proportion to the magnitude of the received IR light. This can be used when the presence or absence of an object is required to be detected, before any further task or analysis is carried out. IR distance sensor is very efficient and cost-effective for this purpose.

3.4.6 ELECTROGONIOMETER

Electrogoniometer is a device used for measuring joint angles. Electrogoniometer continuously measures joint angles and is ideal to measure dynamic movements. It is extremely precise as it is mostly used to determine deformities in patients. The readings can be displayed real time as well as be stored to create a dataset.

For Electrogoniometers, the following three types of devices are mainly used:

1. **Optoelectronic systems:** Video systems are used to track bright markers placed at various locations. These markers can be IR light LEDs or solid shapes of reflective tape. The vertical and horizontal coordinates are tracked of each markers, and then the data are further processed. Figure 3.11 depicts the optoelectronic sensors at three different positions in different angles.

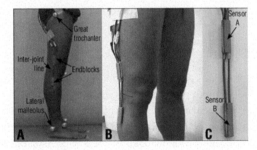

Figure 3.11 Optoelectronic sensors at three different positions

2. **Potentiometers:** In comparison with the traditional goniometer, a potentiometer is positioned over the centre of rotation of the joint being monitored. When motion occurs at the joint, an electrical output from the potentiometer provides a continuous record of the angle present at the joint. Electrical resistance from the potentiometer can be used to determine the angle between the joints. Figure 3.12 shows a potentiometer-type electrogoniometer.

3. **Strain gauges:** These are commonly known as flexible electrogoniometers and are also the most popular type. The strain gauge mechanism is housed inside the spring, which changes its electrical resistance proportionally to the change in angle between the plastic end blocks' longitudinal axes. Figure 3.13 shows a strain gauge-based electrogoniometer.

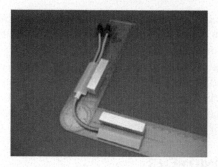

Figure 3.12   Potentiometer-type electrogoniometer

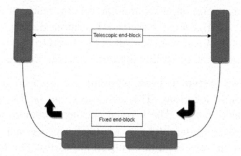

Figure 3.13   Strain gauge-based electrogoniometer

3.5   FALL DETECTION

This section consists of one of the most important and widely used applications of posture detection. Fall detection is one of the main problem especially for older people due to their poor physical fitness. If the old people fell down, then it would be difficult for them to request help. Internet of Things (IoT) and network sensors make it possible to overcome this problem. Using IoT and sensor network, a system can be developed which will be able to detect the falling incident of a person and report it to the healthcare department soonest possible.

3.5.1   SYSTEM DESIGN AND WORKFLOW

Tang et al. [74] proposed the fall detection system for elderly. Figure 3.14 describes the architecture of the proposed system for elderly people. The following workflow of the proposed system has been described by the authors:

1. Falling detection devices like sensors will be worn by elderly people on their wrist or waist.

2. The embedded algorithm will run by a sensor device, and it will detect the geographic location and body measures of the person.

3. If the body position detected by the sensor device is in falling mode, the system-embedded alarm will be triggered.

4. If the alarm is triggered by mistake (false positive), the user can reset the alarm by clicking on the reset button.

5. If the alarm is not cancelled within 15 seconds, then an emergency SMS with the user's geographic location will be sent to the contact person.

6. After sending the SMS, the system will automatically reset the alarm to its original condition.

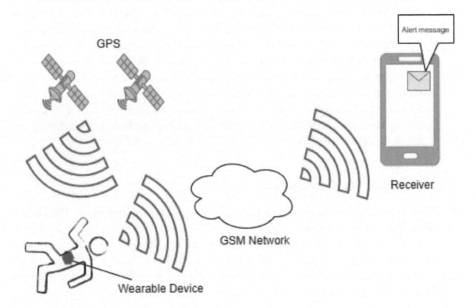

Figure 3.14   Architecture of the system [75]

3.5.2 FALL DETECTION SYSTEM

There are mainly two types of existing system for fall detection [76]:

1. **Wearable System:** In a wearable system, the sensor is embedded within the wearable device worn by the subject in order to detect the fall detection. The sensor-based system consists of an accelerometer, gyroscope and magnetometer which are placed on the subject/person to detect the changes in acceleration, position, the plane of motion or body measure. Other parameters that are monitored by the wearable device-based system are electrocardiogram (ECG), oxygen saturation of blood and heart rate variability (HRV). The data reported

by sensors are then passed to a ML algorithm or checked against a threshold value to classify and detect fall [77].

Wearable systems are usually less expensive, have low power consumption and are small in size, which makes them more convenient to use and easily affordable. Most of the wearable devices are usually in bent form, which can be worn around the wrist or thigh. In smartphone-based devices, sensors are embedded within the smartphones, and when the user carries their smartphone with them, then the smartphone can detect the fall. [78].

2. **Non-wearable System:** The non-wearable system does not include an embedded system that is worn by people. These include cameras, pressure sensors and acoustic sensors which are placed in the subject's normal environment [76]. The non-wearable system does not perform any parameter evaluation; instead it uses an image or video processing captured by the camera to detect the fall. Machine algorithms are applied to the captured image by applying image processing. Generally, convolutional neural networks are trained on different datasets of images to get more accuracy [77]. The non-wearable system provides more accurate details in abnormal conditions via images or video. However, they are more expensive, take more time in processing and are computationally intensive.

3.5.3 DESIGN COMPONENTS

Both hardware and software components are necessary for fall detection. The sensor-based device, microcontroller, comes in the category of hardware which is used to measure the body position and motion and communication with the software system to send out an emergency SMS if falling is detected. If an alarm is triggered by the sensor for 15 seconds, only then the message will be sent to the ambulance. Possible hardware and programming languages may be considered as follows:

a) **Arduino UNO and GPRS:** As described in [74], Arduino UNO and GPRS shield are used as the hardware components. Arduino UNO is an open-source microcontroller board based on the Microchip ATmega328P microcontroller and developed by Arduino. It has 20 I/O pins of which six can be used as analogue inputs and six can be used as PWM outputs, one USB connector, a power jack, reset button, ceramic resonator and an ICSP header. Connection of the USB cable to the computer is required to load a program in Arduino.

GPRS is compatible with Arduino UNO and is based on the SIM900 module from SIMCOM. GSM cell phone network in GPRS shields provides the way to communicate it. By sending AT commands via UART, the GPRS shield allows sending SMS, MMS, audio and GPRS. The GPRS shield also has 12 GPIOs, two PWMs and one ADC. The default setting for the shield UART is 19200 bps 8-N-1 and can be changed by AT commands. A diagram of SIMCOM SIM900 GSM GPRS shield development board is shown in Figure 3.15.

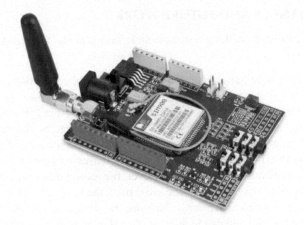

Figure 3.15   Diagram of SIMCOM SIM900 GSM GPRS shield development board [74]

b) **Programming Language Used:** The Arduino IDE supports the languages C and C++ using rules of code structuring [74]. The Arduino IDE already has a software library from wiring projects. Two basic functions are required to write the code, one for starting the sketch and the other for the main program loop. The *avrdude* program in the *Arduino IDE* is used to convert the executable code into a text file in hexadecimal encoding. With the help of the loader program, the text file is loaded in the *Arduino* board. The setup() function is called once, and the loop() function is called repeatedly until the board is reset.

3.5.4   ALGORITHM DESIGN

In fall alarm system, algorithm is mainly based on sum threshold value of acceleration and rotational angle. When fall happens, collision between the body and ground produces a peak value at sum acceleration **a**. Here magnitude of **a** represents the three-axes value of accelerometer. For the first step, system uses sum acceleration to detect high-intensity movement. However, jumping and sitting also produce peak value, so additional feature may be required for the detection.

The second feature is an angle which can be calculated by acceleration measurements to calculate the rotational angle in a three-dimensional space by separating the gravity component before and after fall. When the device is mounted on the elderly wrist or waist, it will record the g value while the person is standing. After measuring all the three different axes, the sum acceleration $|a|$ will be calculated. When elderly fall in real, the acceleration will reach its peak value, which is greater than the threshold value, i.e. $|a| \geq a_{threshold}$ [75]

3.6 CHALLENGES AND FUTURE WORK

In this section, various challenges and possible future works that can be done in this area are discussed.

1. Selection of right transmission interval and data collection that is accurate for a specific purpose is a challenging problem. It depends on the type of considered sensor, and the range varies in wired and wireless sensors. For instance, while collecting the knee data of a person, it is required that the data are transmitted after a regular fixed interval of time (400–500 ms) in the case of wired sensors. Selecting the right transmission interval increases accuracy while training the collected data on a ML model. However, bigger the time interval, more is the chances of the loss of data. At the same time, the lesser the interval, the system will be overloaded. Therefore, selecting the time interval which best fits for considered model and can handle the data flow is very important.

2. While collecting data from multiple sensors, data collection rate may get affected. Due to this, the sensor may start reading wrong data, which affects data quality. Either use of multiple sensors needs to be avoided or there is a need to write a program that works on a particular interval of time to collect that data.

3. Sensor drift is another challenging problem with time-sensitivity of sensors insensate. It means if one sensor is used for a very long time then it is possible that its reading starts to tilt and deviate. Therefore, either changing the sensor after a certain period of time is necessary or algorithm may be designed to tackle the sensor drift.

4. After collecting huge data, it becomes complex to find the interdependency between the different datasets and finding the desired relationship among them. Even if sometimes the relationship can be found between the datasets, it is possible that it would be changed for the different interval or property. For instance, let there exist a dataset of a male in different position and there is a relation between them such that all healthy people have almost the same reading of x, y and z-axis. However, it may be possible that for the females, this doesn't satisfy. Therefore, more data will be needed to get the desired result.

5. In a fall detection, it is necessary that the system works accurately and triggers the alarm within the time. Designing instruments that can prevent fall detection are also a very important factor.

3.7 CONCLUSIONS

The study of human posture has many applications. There are different types of sensors which can be used to collect the human posture data. These data are then used for the classification of a posture as a healthy or unhealthy one using ML techniques. Once the model is trained, the data will be classified in real time after sending it to the model using WiFi. In this chapter, an introduction to human posture recognition using IoT networks is provided. Further, the chapter also summarized the underlying sensor technology that is used in IoT networks involved in human posture detection. This chapter will help in understanding the sensors such that their selection for different situations will be easier. Still, lots of research is going on in this area. This chapter also gave insight into possible future works that can be done for achieving better results.

4 Application of Machine Intelligence in IoT-Enabled Healthcare Monitoring Systems: A Case Study-Based Approach

Amartya Chakraborty, Subhrangshu Adhikary,
Arindam Ghosh and Partha Sarathi Paul

CONTENTS

DOI: 10.1201/9781003239895-4

4.1 INTRODUCTION

The significant advancements in medical science and healthcare have contributed to
the increase in average life expectancy of citizens of most developed and developing
countries. However, there is a growing demand for effective and affordable healthcare solutions that can cater to the needs of people from different social and economic
strata of the society. On the other hand, the technological enrichment obtained with
the implementation of Internet of Things (IoT) in different domains of human life
has been witnessed for the last few decades. This has led to an era of smart devices,
applications and services – all of which leverage the pre-existing infrastructure of
interconnected devices over a network.

The traditional concept of the internet consists of communicating humans, and
the same is based on the steady advancements of digital communication techniques.
This very internet is also the basis of IoT [79], with the distinction that all natural and
man-made objects can be made to communicate over the network. This differs from
the use of the internet by humans. Human beings can observe their surroundings or
situations, analyse and extract information and express themselves using recognized
set of semantics or language structures to other human beings. In the case of objects or 'things', these virtues do not come naturally. The sensors and actuators play
the crucial role of 'observing' the surroundings or environment of an object; the observations come in the form of sensory data in certain accepted format [80]. These
electronic devices are driven by voltage changes, which are regulated by the microcontrollers [81] (or the microprocessors [82], as the case may be) in their internal
circuitry depending on their system requirements. In case a microcontroller is used,
the data is then transmitted over a network utilizing technologies like Bluetooth [83],
Wi-Fi [84] or the GSM [85]. On the contrary, the microprocessor-based systems are
inherently capable of data analysis and optionally transmit data using the available
communication techniques. In general, the data acquired by these sensors and transmitted to a processing device is then analysed. This sensory data, by nature, consists
of sensor readings in temporal sequences. The underlying patterns a.k.a. features of
the data are extracted by using the temporal, statistical or frequency domain signal
processing techniques and computations to generate the representative information
for different types of events in the sensor environment. These features are then fed to
suitable machine learning algorithms that learn from the variance of features and corresponding event labels. These algorithms then predict or determine the occurrence
of the event from another set of features from a different data pool. In general, the
above framework drives most of the IoT-Based applications in this era of smart technologies. This general three-layer IoT framework is portrayed in Figure 4.1 where
the individual layers and their functionalities are illustrated. The framework shown
may be adapted towards the development of smart systems in various avenues of
human life.

The development of IoT-enabled applications catering to various human requirements is fuelled by rigorous research in different fields of study. The advent of internet of healthcare things (IoHT) is one such rich domain of research. The above
field of research utilizes the cost-effective sensing setups with the IoT framework

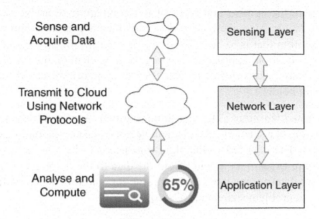

Figure 4.1   General framework of a three-layer IoT-Based system

towards augmenting the field of healthcare and health monitoring. IoHT applications aim to provide affordable healthcare infrastructure, including feasible remote monitoring and even real-time monitoring capabilities. This entails the monitoring of the elderly in indoor environments and affordable healthcare for poverty-stricken or disaster-affected citizens in remote locations [86]. The adaptation of computationally efficient learning techniques also enables the timely and accurate detection and prediction of diseases and aids in the development of medical treatments and drugs for new diseases and health disorders.

4.2   CLASSIFICATION OF MACHINE INTELLIGENCE IN IOT-ENABLED HEALTHCARE SYSTEMS

Smart wearable systems empowered by IoT are able to monitor and capture health-related events in a continuous manner. Such events may range from changes in pulse rate and sweat secretion to mental stress and depression; some of these events may lead to critical health issues such as heart attack or suicide. Given the understanding that every such set of events culminates in an adverse health problem, it is crucial to correctly determine the set of 'meaningful connections' between said events and their effect on health. These 'connections' are best expressed statistically, and researchers have focused for decades on the design of efficient algorithms to derive such connections. Based on several categories of mathematical logic, such algorithms look for hidden patterns in continuous streams of data that are known to lead to particular consequences. These algorithms are thus said to 'learn' from input–output sequences (training). The knowledge gained by a machine that utilizes such algorithms can be generalized to represent the underlying relation between events and outcomes (classifier). This generalization can further be utilized to analyse newer sets of data and determine cause, course or treatment in the early stages of a health problem (classification). Given the huge variation in types of data associated with health-related event detection, the number and types of IoT-compatible wearable sensors are also an important factor. Also, the type of data is elementary in determining the machine learning algorithm that is to be utilized by the smart healthcare system. The 'learning' and 'classification' approaches are largely dependent on the problem statement. Some of the main categories of machine learning algorithm-based models are discussed in brief below:

a) *Supervised learning:* The algorithm learns from a set of 'training' examples consisting of a set of events (element vectors) and corresponding consequences (labels). The data fed to the algorithm needs to be labelled in order for the algorithm to learn a mapping from the data to the output. This intelligence is used for determining the 'class' or value for unknown sets of data gathered for the same problem statement [87, 88].

b) *Unsupervised learning:* Here the algorithm is tasked to determine the different categories or clusters that are represented by the training data. Armed with this knowledge, unseen data patterns are then classified into specific clusters [89, 90].

c) *Semi-supervised learning:* In some critical problems, there are only a few sets of training data whose consequences are recorded, i.e. for which ground truth information is available. In such cases, the algorithm utilizes both the labelled and unlabelled element vectors and predicts consequences on unknown data thereafter [91, 92].

d) *Transfer learning:* There may exist particular problems where the availability of ground truth information and consequently labelled element vectors is rare or unfeasible. As a result, the classification algorithm fails to appropriately learn from the sparsely represented data. In such cases, the data and corresponding knowledge from a related domain may be utilized for determining the classes in the sparsely labelled problem statement [93, 94].

. Further in this part of the chapter, the authors undertake a comprehensive study of the widely used supervised learning algorithms in terms of their working principles, health issues identified as per state-of-the-art research and remarks related to their applicability in determining health issues. A tabular summary is also illustrated for each of the learning techniques discussed in this section, where each work is defined in terms of its objective(s), sensors or data, and remarks regarding its performance or shortcoming.

4.2.1 NON-PROBABILISTIC HYPERPLANE-BASED CLASSIFIERS

The concept of 'hyperplane' for determining the class of new data points in an n-dimensional space is utilized in the algorithm known as support vector machine (SVM) [95]. It is a supervised learning algorithm that utilizes the recorded ground truth information to learn the event-to-consequence mapping from the processed data. Given an element vector consisting of n features, the algorithm determines the 'optimal separation hyperplane' that can be used to prominently distinguish between the different classes of data points. For this purpose, the data elements that are closer to the proposed hyperplane are used to rectify its position in order to maximize the margin of separation, called the support vectors. This is illustrated in the two sub-parts of Figure 4.2 for a two-class problem. The left-side sub-figure illustrates how numerous hyperplanes of separation are possible, and the right-side sub-figure illustrates how with the support of the closest data points an optimal hyperplane is determined. In these illustrations, the two classes of data are represented with triangles and circles, and the support vectors are shaded in black. In the following section, a brief discussion of the use of SVM in wearable sensor–based healthcare systems in state-of-the-art research is undertaken.

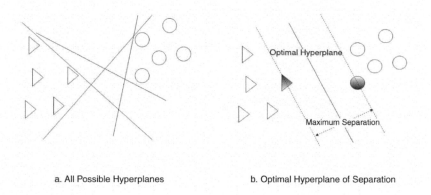

a. All Possible Hyperplanes   b. Optimal Hyperplane of Separation

Figure 4.2 Illustration of SVM working; the set of all possible hyperplanes is shown in the left, and the optimal separating hyperplane is given in the right.

In the early stages of IoHT-based research, patients who were at the risk of developing mental issues such as early or late stage psychosis were identified using SVM as the algorithm of choice on processed MRI images [96] with classification efficiency between 86% and 93% in different cases. Similarly, accelerometer-based human motion data with a trained SVM classifier was used to determine the severity of symptoms related to Parkinson's disease [97]. Error rates were reduced from 6% to 1.2% by teaching the classifier with more features based on the accelerometer data. Electrocardiogram (ECG) signals were utilized by the SVM algorithm to monitor and determine episodes of obstructive sleep apnoea [98] with a high accuracy of about 90%. Stress recognition based on several novel factors was undertaken using SVM classifier on processed sensor, phone usage and survey data [99]. The system reported over 75% accuracy in terms of classification performance. Drowsiness detection system based on wearable sensor data such as heart rate and stress level was deployed for accident prevention and achieved over 98% accuracy when the features were classified using the SVM algorithm [100]. Thus, it can be seen that different types of image and sensor data are usable by the SVM algorithm to identify

Table 4.1
Summary of Contemporary Research in IoHT Using SVM

Reference	Objective	Sensor Used/Type of Data	Remarks
Koutsouleris et al. [96]	Detection of early-stage psychosis	MRI images	83–96% in different cases
Patel et al. [97]	Determine Parkinson's disease symptom severity	Accelerometer data	1.2% error rate in best case
Bsoul et al. [98]	Detection of obstructive sleep apnoea	ECG signals	90% accuracy
Leng at al. [100]	Drowsiness detection	Heart rate and stress level	98% accuracy
Sano et al. [99]	Stress recognition	Survey and phone usage data	75% accuracy

both physical and mental abnormalities associated with human health. Using the predetermined set of features, these works are listed in Table 4.1.

4.2.2   PROBABILISTIC CLASSIFIERS

This type of supervised learning algorithm determines the probability distribution over a set of known classes for a newly observed data value. Based on the 'naive' assumption that the features in training data are independent of each other, this type of supervised learning algorithm makes use of the *Bayes' theorem*. This is known as the *Naive Bayes algorithm* [101]. The Bayes' theorem is concerned with determining the probability of occurrence of any event, given the probability of another event that has already occurred. This understanding is used for determining the class label of any unknown data point, when the conditional probabilities of known inputs are available and the output is also known. Such a technique finds use particularly in the case of large data sets. The theorem, when applied to a set of feature variables $x_1, x_2, x_3, \cdots x_n$ belonging to feature vector X and a class label y, is stated as

$$P(y|X) = \frac{P(X|y) \cdot P(y)}{P(X)} \tag{4.1}$$

Next, the factor of independence among feature variables is introduced, which changes the Equation (4.1) to

$$P(y|x_1, x_2, \cdots, x_n) = \frac{P(x_1|y) \cdot P(x_2|y) \cdots P(x_n|y) \cdot P(y)}{P(x_1) \cdot P(x_2) \cdots P(x_n)} \tag{4.2}$$

For a given set of training data, the values of $P(x_1), P(x_2), \cdots P(x_n)$ are constant, and thus the Equation (4.2) is further modified to

$$P(y|x_1, x_2, \cdots, x_n) \propto P(x_1|y) \cdot P(x_2|y) \cdots P(x_n|y) \cdot P(y) \tag{4.3}$$

In order to create a corresponding classifier model, commonly referred to as the *Naive Bayes Classifier* model, the probability of a known set of inputs is calculated for all possible values of class label y, and the output with the maximum probability value is picked as the predicted class. This classification algorithm is regularly used for solving healthcare related problems; some state-of-the-art works are discussed below.

The early usage of ECG, respiration, skin conductance and electromyogram (EMG)-based features to classify stress and non-stress situations based on a set of healthy subjects was seen in the work of Wijsman et al. [102]. The Naive Bayes classifier was utilized to achieve a minimum error rate of 0.2 when classified using selected features. The detection of mental conditions in a set of 12 patients with bipolar disorder was conducted with the same classification approach [103]. Smartphone-based inertial sensor and Global Positioning System (GPS) sensor data was utilized for the detection of mental state and state change. A state recognition accuracy of over 76% was achieved by the researchers, with over 97% recall in the detection of state changes. In a very similar research by the authors of the former work [104], an 800-day-long data set gathered from ten participants affected by bipolar disorder was gathered to trace 17 different changes in their mental state. In this work, Naive Bayes classifier was successfully able to identify the mental states with about 80% accuracy and state changes with a recall of 94%. A different type of work [105] also utilized smartphone-based inertial sensors for the detection of stress levels in 30 working professionals. The detection of low, moderate and high stress was achieved with an accuracy of 71% using the Naive Bayes algorithm. The application of this probabilistic approach can be seen in classifying sensor data towards the recognition of mental disorders. In healthcare-related applications, the Naive Bayes algorithm has been mainly used for the classification of EMG, IMU or GPS sensor data in resolving problems related to mental stress and disorders. These are listed parametrically in Table 4.2.

4.2.3 FEATURE DISTANCE-BASED CLASSIFIERS

The use of distance metrics for the identification of the class of a given data point is noted in a simplistic supervised algorithm, called the *k-nearest neighbours (kNN)*

Table 4.2

Summary of Contemporary Research in IoHT Using Naive Bayes

Reference	Objective	Sensor Used/Type of Data	Remarks
Wijsman et al. [102]	Detection of stress vs. non-stress	ECG, respiration, skin conductance and EMG	Error rate of 0.2
Gruenerbl et al. [103]	Detection of mental state change in patients with bipolar disorder	Smartphone IMU and GPS data	Over 76% accuracy
Grunerbl et al. [104]	Detection of 17 different mental state changes in patients with bipolar disorder	Smartphone IMU and GPS data	Over 80% accuracy
Garcia et al. [105]	Detection of stress levels	Smartphone IMU sensor data	71% accuracy

classifier [106]. It is easier to interpret and widely used in classification and regression problems. The algorithm uses training data only at the time of classification and attempts to identify the similarity between the known and the new data. This similarity is determined in terms of a distance-based metric, say the Euclidean distance. The class which has the most representation in the neighbourhood of k-nearest data points is determined as the class of the new data point that is to be classified. This concept is explained with the help of a simple example in Figure 4.3.

As seen in the illustration, the stars and suns represent the known data points in the training set. Given a new data value, marked as X, the kNN classifier tries to determine the class this new value belongs to, based on the neighbours in its proximity. For instance, when the number of neighbours is set to $k = 3$, the neighbourhood consists of two stars and one sun. Accordingly, the kNN classifier will determine that the unclassified data value belongs to the class of stars. However, this prediction is not ultimate, as any change in the value of k may lead to a different prediction. This is seen when the number of neighbours is set to $k = 7$. The number of suns ($= 4$) in this case exceeds the number of stars ($= 3$), and so the algorithm predicts that the unclassified value X belongs to the class of suns. This contradicts the prediction

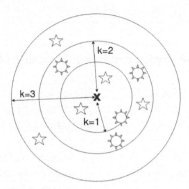

Figure 4.3   Illustration of the kNN algorithm; here k denotes the number of neighbours to be considered while determining the class of the unknown data.

with $k = 3$ neighbours discussed earlier. Again, if the number of neighbours is set to $k = 9$, the class prediction changes to stars. Thus, it is also implied that the choice of an optimal value of k is crucial for any classification problem to be solved.

An early example of the usage of kNN in healthcare solution is the work by Lan et al. where the cognitive state of subjects while performing different types of activities was identified from electroencephalography (EEG) signals [107]. The system showed a classification capability with about 80% accuracy with the use of kNN classifier model. The work by Sano et al. [99] determined novel features from accelerometer, skin conductance and phone usage data along with surveys to identify stress in a group of healthy subjects. The kNN algorithm performed with an accuracy as high as 75%. A novel work utilized redundancy graph–based feature selection on IMU data to identify transitions between different body postures and activities [108]. The system performed with an accuracy of 97% by using the kNN classifier. Similarly, IMU data was gathered to identify similar gait in volunteers by gathering different types of walking data. On an average, the system performed with about 93% accuracy based on the decision of the kNN classifier [109]. Table 4.3 lists these works in terms of the preset parameters relevant to our study.

4.2.4   BIOLOGICALLY INSPIRED CLASSIFIERS

The artificial neural networks (ANNs) [110], also simply called as neural networks, are decision-making models loosely based on the biological neural systems of human brains. An animal's nervous system essentially consists of biological neurons connected via synapses that convey signals. In much the same way, ANNs consist of artificial nodes or neurons that are capable of receiving and sending signals to other connected neurons. The signals in this case are simply real numbers, and the output of a particular neuron is computed using pre-defined functions on all inputs at that neuron. Inspired by the biological nervous system, the ANNs are thus capable of receiving and pre-processing, processing and computing, and finally providing the

Table 4.3
Summary of Contemporary Research in IoHT Using kNN

Reference	Objective	Sensor Used/Type of Data	Remarks
Sano et al. [99]	Stress identification	Accelerometer, skin conductance and phone usage	75% accuracy
Ghasemzadeh et al. [108]	Identify body posture transitions	IMU data	97% accuracy
Ngo et al. [109]	Identifying similar gait	IMU data	93% accuracy
Lan et al. [107]	Identifying cognitive state of subjects while performing different activities	EEG signals	80% accuracy

outputs in an interpretable form to aid decision-making. The overview of a simple neural network is shown in Figure 4.4 which illustrates the presence of three types of layers in a typical neural network – one input layer, n number of hidden layers and one output layer. The input layer is tasked with communicating with the outside world and receiving the inputs. The hidden layer(s) transforms the input in such a way that they represent underlying information in the input data. This information

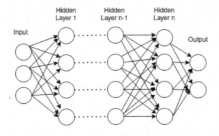

Figure 4.4   General structure of an artificial neural network with n hidden layers

is used by the output layer towards solving the given problem. The number of input neurons, hidden layers (and neurons in each hidden layer) and output neurons varies depending on input data characteristics and problem requirements.

The general structure of a neuron is shown in Figure 4.5. Each neuron in the network takes a set of inputs $x_1, x_2, \cdots x_n$ with corresponding weights w_{ij}, multiplies them and finally sums them up. The 'bias' value is augmented to the sum, and a special 'activation function' $f()$ is applied to the result. This introduces non-linearity in the output from the neuron, which is passed onto all the neurons that are further connected.

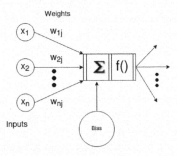

Figure 4.5   General structure of a neuron

There are different types of neural network architectures that researchers have developed over the years. Almost all of the advanced architectures are applied in solving healthcare-related decision-making problems, and some of these state-of-the-art works are discussed in the following section.

Over the years, different variations of neural networks have been utilized by researchers for solving different types of healthcare-related problems. The radial basis function (RBF)-based neural network system was developed by Wu et al. [111]. Data gathered from Parkinson's disease patients using deep brain electrodes was classified to predict tremors with an accuracy of 90%. The convolutional neural network (CNN)-based classifiers were used to detect five different types of arrhythmia in ECG data with an overall accuracy of 99% [112]. Another special type of network, called the probabilistic neural network, was used to identify seven types of arrhythmia and normal heart beat with a 99% accuracy rate [87]. A set of frequency domain features extracted from slices of brain image data was used for training ANN [113]. The system was able to differentiate between pathological and healthy brain images with accuracy over 99% in the best case. The auto-encoder features were extracted using ANN model from noisy speech data and trained with SVM classifier for emotion recognition [114]. Also, Alzheimer's disease detection was carried out using deep belief network (DBN)-based neural network classifier with an accuracy of 87.5% [88]. The possibility of adverse events in patients admitted to the ICU was detected using ANNs [115]. For learning, the system used the patient's vital statistics and lab reports and predicted the possibility of emergency within 4 hours with 78% positive prediction rate.

Normal and accident-affected cerebral vascular regions were identified from computer tomographic (CT) images by RBF-based neural network [116] with high sensitivity and specificity of about 97%. A CNN model was utilized for the recognition of benign from malignant glands with a high F1-score of 90% [117]. The work by Huang et al. [118] reduced the error rate in comparison with state-of-the-art works for the problem of foetal cardiac screening from 3D video data. The angle and location of the heart were successfully determined with a minimized error rate of about 21% using ANN model. The detection of loss of hearing in patients suffering from sensorineural hearing loss was undertaken by [119]. The ANN model was used to classify features extracted from brain tissue MRI images, and the system performed with 95% accuracy. The extraction of features and feature reduction were carried out with DBN towards the identification of genes related to glioblastoma (a form of brain tumour) in an unsupervised classification problem [120].

A CNN model was proposed to identify four types of interstitial lung disease and healthy lungs from CT scan image slices [121]. The system achieved a high area under the curve (AUC) score of 0.99. The detection of malignant tissue from real-time surgical video feed was reported by [122] with a remarkable maximum delay of 77 seconds! A long short-term memory (LSTM)-based neural network classifier working with electronic patient records was capable of diagnosing diabetes with an accuracy of 96% while predicting the progress in Parkinson's disease also with re-markable accuracy [123]. In a similar work, a volumetric data set of ECG recordings was used for the recognition of 12 classes of arrhythmia [124]. The system reported an F1-score of 81% in comparison with the 75% score by cardiologists!

Some of the state-of-the-art works are listed in Tables 4.3 and 4.4. It is obvious that in comparison with the conventional machine learning algorithms, ANN-based models and their variations have been preferred by researchers in dealing with different complex problems in IoT-Based healthcare. A wide range of data can be handled by such networks, and their functionality also finds application in feature reduction for other supervised, semi-supervised or unsupervised classification algorithms.

4.3   CASE STUDY: WALKING DEFECT DETECTION USING SMARTPHONE DATA

In the present section of the chapter, the usage of smartphone sensors as an implementation of an IoT device to study gait is discussed and a case study is presented. We narrate state-of-the-art research works performed to study gait using machine learning and finally illustrate the usage of machine learning to detect the walking defects.

4.3.1   GAIT, SMARTPHONE SENSORS AND THE USE OF MACHINE LEARNING TO DETECT WALKING DEFECTS

The study behind the mechanics of walk is called gait. Different neuro-skeletal disorders impact the gait of a human being. Corresponding to neurological disorders, there are eight types of gaits, viz. *hemiplegic, spastic diplegic, neuropathic, myopathic,*

Table 4.4
Summary of Contemporary Research in IoHT Using Different Types of ANNs

Reference	Objective	Sensor Used/Type of Data	Variation of Neural Network	Remarks
Wu et al. [111]	Prediction of tremor in Parkinson's disease patients	Deep brain electrode data	Radial basis function (RBF)	90% accuracy
Krizhevsky et al. [112]	Detection of five types of arrhythmia	ECG data	Convolutional neural network (CNN)	99% accuracy
Wang et al. [87]	Detection of seven types of arrhythmia and normal heart beat	ECG data	Probabilistic neural network	99% accuracy
Zhang et al. [113]	Detection of pathological vs. healthy brain	Slices of brain image data	Artificial neural network	99% accuracy
Zhang et al. [114]	Emotion recognition	Noisy speech data	Artificial neural network	Auto-encoder features extracted
Hu et al. [88]	Alzheimer's disease detection	MRI image data	Deep belief network	87.5% accuracy
Hu et al. [115]	Detection of adverse events in ICU-admitted patients, predicted possibility of emergency within 4 hours	Patient's vital statistics and lab reports	Artificial neural network	78% positive prediction rate
Ruano et al. [116]	Detection of normal and accident-affected cerebral vascular regions	Computer tomographic (CT) images	Radial basis function (RBF)	97% sensitivity and specificity
Chen et al. [117]	Identification of benign from malignant glands	Histology images	Convolutional neural network (CNN)	90% F1 score
Huang et al. [118]	Foetal cardiac screening	3D video data	Artificial neural network	Error rate reduced to 21%
Wang et al. [119]	Detection of hearing loss	MRI image data	Artificial neural network	95% accuracy
Young et al. [120]	Identification of glioblastoma-related genes	Gene expression data	Deep belief network	Feature extraction and reduction
Gao et al. [121]	Detection of four types of interstitial lung disease and healthy lungs	Computer tomographic (CT) images	Convolutional neural network (CNN)	AUC score of 99%
Salvador et al. [122]	Malignant tissue identification	Surgical video feed (real time)	Artificial neural network	Maximum delay of only 77 seconds
Baytas et al. [123]	Diabetes prediction and progress in Parkinson's disease	Electronic patient records	Long short-term memory (LSTM) network	96% accuracy
Rajpurkar et al. [124]	Detection of 12 classes of arrhythmia	60,000 ECG records	Convolutional neural network (CNN)	81% F1 score
Deperlioglu et al. [125]	Detection of different heart diseases	Heart sound data sets	Auto-encoder deep neural network	96% accuracy
Adhikary et al. [126]	Detection of COVID-19 from chest X-ray	X-ray image data	Convolution neural network (CNN)	95.02% accuracy
Abdel et al. [127]	Activity recognition	HAR data sets	Long short-term memory (LSTM) network	98.9% accuracy
Khamparia et al. [128]	Detection of cervical cancer cells	Pap smear images	Convolutional neural network (CNN)	97.8% F1 score

Parkinsonian, choreiform, ataxic (cerebellar) and *sensory*. Other conditions like *osteoarthritis*, injury, etc., also contribute towards defective gait. Therefore, monitoring of walking mechanics is of prior importance to detect several underlying conditions [129]. To monitor gait, a variety of techniques can be used, which include applying video surveillance, developing specialized environments or using wearable sensors. Video surveillance is very popular for this purpose as it can be easily deployed in a wide range of environments [130]. However, this comes with a high computational cost, since, to process a large number of video frames, the deep learning models need to be trained with a high volume of manually processed training data and need to be trained for a large number of iterations. After this, the frames need to be arranged in time series to learn the sequence of changes in the movements corresponding to different abnormalities. Apart from the high computational costs, the detection accuracy of this process is lower compared to wearable sensors and specialized environment-sensing approaches, as different camera angles may require retraining of the data, thus increasing the computational challenges [131]. Developing specialized environments works excellent in monitoring gait as these types of environments are built with a combination of pressure sensors on the path or other movement-capturing sensors [132]. This requires significantly less computational power as there are only fixed orientation and position of sensors compared to one another and it does not require much calibration of the sensors. However, the challenges with this type are that it is not portable and have high setup and maintenance cost. Finally, wearable sensors are nowadays very popular as they are portable, require less computational complexity and low setup and maintenance cost [133]. This approach includes pressure sensors embedded within shoes, accelerometer or gyroscopes attached in legs, hands, etc. The present case study demonstrates the usage of smartphone-embedded motion sensors to study gait, as an inexpensive and widely available alternative to study walking defects remotely utilizing machine learning and deep learning algorithms [134]. Figure 4.6 shows the comparison of normal and defective walk patterns based on tri-axial accelerometer and tri-axial gyroscope. Here

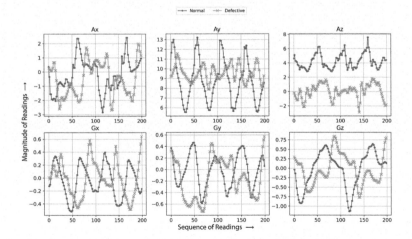

Figure 4.6 Comparison of normal and defective walk pattern based on tri-axial accelerometer and tri-axial gyroscope

blue lines denote normal walk signatures, and orange lines denote defective ones. Readings from A_y show one of the most distinct features as they show the displacement from the ground while walking. A regular normal pattern has a deviation from around 5.5 to 13 ms^{-2}; however, the defective restricted gait ranges from 8 to 11 ms^{-2}. Another prominently visible difference includes A_z where normal forward acceleration ranges between 3 and 6 ms^{-2} but a defective restricted gait ranges between -2 and 2 ms^{-2}.

4.3.2 WALKING DEFECT DETECTION TECHNIQUE

The walking defects can be detected with different machine learning techniques using smartphone-embedded sensors as discussed in the following text. Figure 4.7 gives an overview of the proposed walking-pattern-monitoring system.

4.3.2.1 Data Collection, Filtering and Pre-Processing

Motion sensors like tri-axial accelerometers and tri-axial gyroscopes are nowadays available in smartphones. Therefore, to track motion, a smartphone with a programmed data collector has been placed on the chest near the sternum of human subjects with consent, affixed with specially prepared belts. With consent from human subjects, we have tracked normal healthy individuals and individuals with walking defects. From both categories, there were ten subjects each. The data has been recorded as A_x, A_y and A_z for the three axes of the accelerometer and G_x, G_y and G_z for the three axes of the gyroscope. The motion signatures are recorded at a rate of 100Hz $\pm$ 1 for about $30-35$ seconds based on the comfort of different subjects having walking defects and environmental circumstances for other subjects. After capturing the motion information, the data is transferred to the remote storage for further analysis. Here, the data has been trimmed for few seconds from start and end which contributes towards the acceleration and deceleration time. Further, in general,

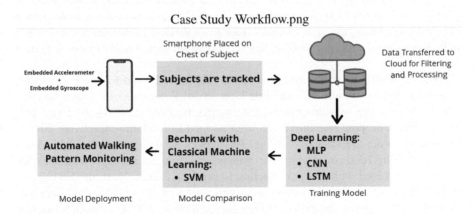

Figure 4.7 Workflow for the walking pattern monitoring system to detect walking defects

machine learning algorithms used in the model tend to work better between the normalized scale of 0 to 1, and therefore, to facilitate this, the data has been min-max scaled to fit within the said range. The data belonging to normal healthy subjects was labelled as 'normal' and for defective subjects was labelled as 'defective'. After this step, all the data was combined into one data set and used for manifold cross-validation towards determining system performance in the experiment.

4.3.2.2 Supervised Deep Learning-Based Classification Model for Gait Anomaly Identification

Deep learning is a subset of machine learning, which works as a series of matrix multiplication operations inspired by the neural communication of the human brain. Three different deep learning techniques have been used in the experiment, viz. multi-layer perceptron (MLP), CNN and LSTM. To observe the performance improvement of deep learning compared to a classical machine learning approach, SVM has been used [135]. The working of SVM is already discussed in Section 4.2.1. In contrast, MLP is the simplest form of deep learning in which several layers of neural networks are stacked over each other. The model is trained to mimic the given outputs by minimizing the error by means of different weight optimizers such as stochastic gradient descent, Adam, etc. There are multiple activation layers such as rectified linear unit (ReLU) , sigmoid, hyperbolic tangent, etc., to introduce non-linearity in the model. Dropouts are used to randomly deactivate different nodes in the network to reduce over-fitting. Other parameters such as L1 and L2 regularizers are often used to regulate over-fitting. CNN is a complex form of MLP where multiple feature extracting layers are used on top of a regular MLP [136]. These feature extraction layers primarily consist of several convolution filters, Gaussian filters, co-occurrence matrices, etc., which are then followed by maxpooling layer to extract the most significant feature among all in order to minimize resource consumption. These are specialized to work with images. However, CNNs can also work excellent with time series data [137]. Lastly, LSTM is a form of recurrent neural network (RNN) which works by keeping some of the learned data in memory variables which are then used during the next epoch in order to facilitate a probabilistic comparison in between the different parts of the data set. These are specialized to work with time series.

The details of the three neural networks' architecture used for the experiments have been given in Figure 4.8. The first layer of MLP consists of a flatten function which converts the two-dimensional data matrix into one-dimensional array. Following this, a dropout rate of 0.2 has been applied to randomly deactivate 20% of the nodes in order to reduce over-fitting. The tensors are then passed through a dense layer containing 1000 nodes which are again passed from a dense layer with one node which is combined with softmax function to produce output. Next, the LSTM network has been built with 16 memory units with a dropout rate of 0.2 passed through a dense layer containing one node and then passed through a RLU activation function to present the output. Finally, the CNN has been built with a one-dimensional convolution layer with 32 feature filters followed by a maxpooling layer with a window

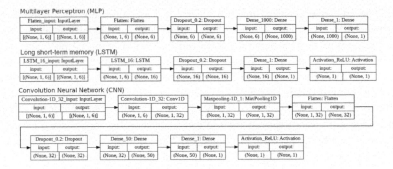

Figure 4.8   The network architecture for the three neural network models

size of 1. The tensors produced from maxpooling are flattened to convert into a one-dimensional array on which a dropout rate of 0.2 has been applied. The results are then passed through two dense layers with 50 nodes and one node, respectively, and finally, the output has been passed through a RLU activation function to produce the results.

4.3.3   PERFORMANCE EVALUATION FOR WALKING DEFECT DETECTION WITH MACHINE LEARNING

The experiment has been conducted on a total of 20 human subjects dividing them into two classes: 'normal walk' and 'defective walk' and recorded in Table 4.5. The data set has been trained with three deep learning models, viz. MLP, CNN

Table 4.5
Performance Comparison of Classical Machine Learning and Three Deep Learning Models in walking Defect Detection System

Metric	SVM	MLP	CNN	LSTM
Accuracy	71.60	84.25	91.61	84.68
Precision	0.71	0.84	0.92	0.85
Recall	0.72	0.84	0.92	0.85
F1-score	0.71	0.84	0.92	0.85
Train Time (s)	93.8	245.8	344.4	304.5
Prediction Time (s)	13.24	0.18	0.22	0.38

and LSTM, and one classical machine learning algorithm, SVM, for the competitive benchmark. It has been observed that CNN has successfully detected walking defects with up to 91.61% accuracy followed by LSTM being 84.68% accurate and MLP being 84.25% accurate. All three deep learning algorithms are considerably better than SVM which has obtained 71.60% accuracy for the overall classification. The reason behind this is that SVM works by creating a hyperplane separating the two classes, but it is difficult to reliably classify complex data without over-fitting or dimensional transformation, which in turn increases the model complexity. Now, MLP gives much better performance than SVM because the model learns by amplifying the features present within the data set, which allows it to establish more complex relationships between the data points. Now, both CNN and LSTM are increments to a regular MLP. Therefore, all properties of MLP are possessed by both CNN and LSTM. In addition, they possess their own signature properties, and therefore these two often tend to perform better than a regular MLP. However, CNN working better than LSTM in our experiment scenario indicates that the feature extraction from the data set works better than following the inherent temporal sequence of data.

Now, for imbalanced data sets where the number of data points in the classes are unequal, other metrics need to be evaluated for a better understanding of the model performance. For these scenarios, metrics like precision, recall and F1-score can be used. In our scenario, all these metrics lie in close proximity, which indicates that there is very little imbalance in our data set. Apart from these, resource optimization could be studied for the different classifier models for determining the system classifier. CNN, though highly accurate, took a very long time to train, about 344.4 sec. to converge, followed by LSTM taking 304.5 sec., MLP with 245.8 sec. and SVM with 93.8 sec. Although SVM worked the fastest here, it cannot be considered fast for larger data sets due to its $O(n^3)$ time complexity, where n is the number of data points. Such a high time complexity makes SVM very slow when the data set size grows. On the other hand, the time complexity of all the three deep learning models discussed here is $O(k)$, where k is the number of iterations till it converges to a global minima of loss. The above makes it grow in time at a linear scale, and therefore for very large data sets, all the above three deep learning algorithms would not have much difference in time consumption. Therefore, considering both detection accuracy and resource consumption aspects, CNN is found to be a good choice for the detection of walking defects.

On a closer investigation of the detection accuracy, the model performances to detect individual classes and their relative difficulty could be understood. From Figure 4.9, it can be observed that the CNN has successfully detected the normal cases with 93.78% detection accuracy, whereas the detection of defective cases was slightly lower with 89.37% detection accuracy. This indicates that there are combinations of gait recordings present within a defective data set which can correlate to a normal walk as well. Compared to other algorithms, CNN is able to detect such patterns much better than the remaining algorithms. LSTM detected normal cases with 87.27% accuracy and defective cases with 82.01% accuracy. MLP has detected the normal cases with 85.76% accuracy, whereas it has detected defective cases with 82.68% accuracy. Finally, it can be noticed that SVM has detected normal cases with

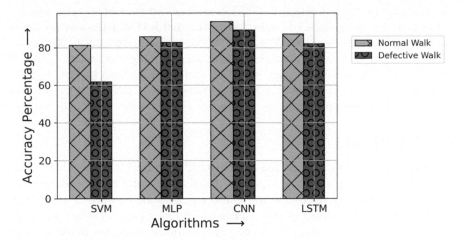

Figure 4.9 Comparison of accuracy for detecting truly normal and truly defective walk cases from gait using different machine learning and deep learning models

81.24% accuracy, whereas it did not perform well to detect defective cases – its detection accuracy for these cases was 61.68%. Therefore, it can be noticed that CNN has been able to detect both normal and defective cases with similar high accuracy, and hence it could safely be used for walking defect detection purpose.

On further exploration, the detection heatmap reveals more information about the performance of each individual class. Figure 4.10 shows the heatmap of all the four models and their corresponding detection of 'true' and 'false' types. It can be noticed that CNN has the highest (48%) normal predictions which are truly normal, the highest (44%) defective predictions which are truly defective, the lowest (5.2%) normal predictions which are actually defective and the lowest (3.2%) defective predictions which are actually normal. On the other hand, SVM has the lowest percentage of true

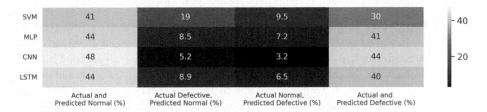

Figure 4.10 Heatmap showing the number of true-positive, false-negative, false-positive and true-negative detections where the colourmap indicates the percentage of cases where lighter colour represents higher number of predictions belonging to that category.

and predicted (41%) and defective (30%) detections and the highest false-negative (19%) and false-positive (9.5%) detections. MLP and LSTM detections lie within similar ranges and in between SVM and CNN detection performances. Therefore, from these results, it could be concluded that deep learning approaches like MLP, CNN and LSTM for defective gait detection works better than classical machine learning like SVM, and within deep learning frameworks, CNN works the best and reliably for the current problem.

4.4 CHALLENGES

The chapter has so far discussed and demonstrated the different learning techniques and their adaptation in IoHT-based research and also illustrated how a walk anomaly detection system can be realized using the IoHT framework. However, it is noteworthy that any such IoT-Based system is prone to different types of issues and faces multiple challenges. In this section, some of the pertinent challenges in the development and deployment of IoT-Based systems are discussed, which require solutions for increasing the adaptability of IoHT systems at large.

1. **Big Data Management**: A large volume of different types of sensor data is generated by sensors in IoT-Based healthcare systems. This big data varies in terms of data format, sampling rate, inherent noise, etc., and the trade-off between these parameters is a rigorous challenge towards the development of a real-time, efficient IoT-Based healthcare system. The adaptation of efficient database systems, energy-efficient connectivity and the involvement of parallel processing should be in focus, while maintaining a sustainable system development cost [138].

2. **Digital Divide**: The technological barrier is another challenge faced by these IoHT-based systems. Often in remote healthcare monitoring systems, the data is captured by patients who are not much aware or comfortable with the usage of sophisticated sensing devices. The interfacing of such deployments should be appropriated such that there is timely data acquisition with minimum intervention by experts. The inclusion of common users' experience towards the development of such systems may ensure their proper utility [139].

3. **Regulatory Frameworks**: As the data gathered consists of various types of medical parameters, a lot of regulatory norms are involved based on territorial or administrative jurisdictions. It is a challenge to develop an acceptable IoHT product that is compatible with the multi-regulatory framework based on different premises. A proper realization of the target areas in terms of geographical or administrative boundaries should be made to increase acceptability of the developed system [140].

4. **Network Reliability**: The IoHT framework is largely dependent on the network layer properties, and the lack of reliability in network conditions is a huge challenge. Especially, in a developing country scenario, the concept of remote healthcare faces a remarkable challenge of developing a network-related

fault-tolerant IoHT framework that may be affordable to the common users. All-inclusive infrastructural development is crucial for the sustenance of an IoHT-enriched ecosystem [141].

5. **Privacy**: The issue of privacy is the most challenging issue in IoHT-based systems. The privacy of different forms of sensitive or insensitive data gathered from human subjects should be ensured in keeping with regulatory norms, the lack of which leads to mistrust and negative perception about such systems. The acquired big data also faces different network security–based challenges when kept in cloud, and more robust security measures must be guaranteed to ensure maximum participation of common masses in IoHT-based implementations [142].

6. **Scalability**: The rapidly rising usage of IoT-enabled systems across the globe is also a major challenge that needs to be addressed promptly. The storage, transmission, network protocol frameworks, etc., that are currently in use need to be scalable to provide support to the inevitable, imminent wave of IoT-enabled devices in a massive network [143].

7. **Energy Efficiency**: The nodes in the IoT systems are usually resource constrained in terms of memory capacity, processing capacity, etc. The larger the network, the more is the energy requirement to drive the IoT-Based system. It is a challenging task to infuse energy efficiency in such an ecosystem. There have been many state-of-the-art systems where energy-efficient data acquisition, data processing and data transmission schemes have been proposed [144].

8. **Maintenance and Upgradation**: The IoT systems generally utilize low-cost sensors and transducers, which have limited service life. In many cases, their sensitivity, range or efficiency may also be affected over time. It is an inherent challenge to regularly monitor, replace or update the existing nodes in any IoT system. The timely and accurate identification of faulty nodes is also a challenging research problem that grows proportional to the adaptation of IoT [145].

The brief study of the aforementioned challenges clearly highlights how there still exist multiple critical issues in the way of a wider deployment and acceptability of such systems. Future research related to IoHT should be directed towards resolving these different challenges that act as hurdles in the way of their development as robust and dependable solutions.

4.5   CONCLUSIONS

The augmentation of IoT in traditional healthcare and health monitoring systems is a vital step towards the development of a smart and affordable medical infrastructure. This chapter highlights this importance by introducing the general IoT framework to the readers, along with some basic algorithms involved in computational intelligence and their usage in state-of-the-art research works. A relevant case study is also included in the later part of the chapter where an IoT-Based healthcare system is designed and tested for the detection of normal vs. abnormal (defective) gait patterns. Last but not the least, some common challenges that require attention for the advent of feasible and acceptable IoHT systems have been discussed in detail. The chapter aims to provide general readers with a basic understanding regarding the inclusion and development of IoT-enabled healthcare systems and will act as a manual for students and researchers willing to work on IoHT applications.

5 Application of Machine Learning in IoHT

Ankit Songara, Pankaj Dhiman and
Summit Bandotra

CONTENTS

5.1 INTRODUCTION

Internet of things (IoT) is one of the rapidly expanding technology which is a network of devices or networks connected together to provide real-time information [146]. Machine learning (ML) is an impactful method for uncovering insights in data from IoT devices. It consists of several procedures that work smartly to enhance different processes like decision-making in a variety of fields, including education, defence, business and the healthcare industry. ML enables IoT to decipher secret patterns in large amounts of data for optimum prediction and recommendation systems [147]. Healthcare has adopted IoT and ML, allowing virtual computers to create medical records, forecast illness diagnosis and, most notably, track patients in real time.

In healthcare field, machine learning approaches use the growing amount of health data generated by the IoT devices to optimize patient outcomes. These methods offer both exciting applications and major challenges. Medical imaging, natural language interpretation of medical records and genetic knowledge are the three primary fields where ML is used. Many of these fields are concerned with diagnosis,

DOI: 10.1201/9781003239895-5

monitoring and estimation. A vast infrastructure of medical devices currently produces data; however, the enabling infrastructure to properly use the data is often lacking. Many formats in which medical records can be found pose several difficulties in data formatting and can increase noise. Descriptive, exploratory, inferential, statistical and causal data processing methods are the most common. An exploratory analysis establishes correlations between variables in a data set, while a descriptive analysis provides summaries of results without explanation. A predictive research aims to quantify the likelihood of an event at the level of a person, whereas an inferential study attempts to quantify the degree to which an observed correlation in a population would hold beyond the sample from which it was derived. Finally, a causal study identifies how changes in one variable cause changes in another. Although a lot of research has been done in numerous fields, healthcare still needs more extensive research. As healthcare-related issues keep on emerging with a rapid rate, there is a need for continuous study to better understand the diseases and come with the most efficient solutions.

5.1.1 A BRIEF OVERVIEW OF INTERNET OF THINGS

According to a survey, by 2025, there will be more than 55 billion IoT devices, 46 billion more than what we had in 2017 (9 billion) [148]. Most industrial IoT giants, such as Google Cloud IoT Edge, Microsoft Azure IoT, Amazon AWS IoT, etc., now support ML for predictive capabilities. When a sensor detects disproportionate heat or vibration inputs, for example it sends out an alarm. If the same sensor is linked to the internet, the information or data it collects can be used to gain additional insights and perform analytics for later use.

As IoT becomes more common and widespread, large numbers of devices and sensors generate massive amount of data, and numerous IoT applications are built to provide users with fine-grained and more precise services [149]. This big data from the IoT devices can additionally be processed and analysed to deliver insights into IoT service providers and consumers.

Many data-driven analytic procedures are used in emerging the IoT applications to efficiently use large IoT sensing data, and AI algorithms have recently been implemented into IoT data analytics procedures. The main components that make up a smart IoT system [150] are a) electrical and mechanical components; b) ports, antennas and protocols; c) sensors, processors, storage and applications; and d) using analytics to train and execute ML models.

The hundreds of millions of devices that are installed at the edge, in homes and workplaces, warehouses, oil fields and agricultural fields, planes and cars, and vehicles – in all the places – are critical to the success of an IoT solution [151]. So, when we talk about IoT information, what exactly do we mean?

5.2 WHAT IS MACHINE LEARNING?

ML and IoT when used with each other can provide informative insights for decision-making, automated responses, etc. [152]. Predicting future trends and detecting anomalies are some of the areas where IoT and ML are being used at a rapid rate. By analysing large amounts of data with sophisticated algorithms, ML can help decode the hidden patterns in IoT data [153]. It may complement or replace manual processes in critical areas with automated systems that use statistically derived behaviour.

ML for IoT is being used by businesses to conduct predictive capabilities on a broad range of use cases, allowing them to gain new insights and advanced automation capabilities. ML can be used for IoT to ingest and turn data into a consistent and uniform format and create a ML model and install it on the cloud, computer and edge. A business can, for example, automate quality inspection and monitoring on its production line, monitor asset behaviour in the field and forecast usage and demand trends using ML procedures.

With enhancements in emerging technologies such as cloud computing, graphics processing unit (GPU) computing and other hardware advancements, artificial intelligence (AI) has achieved great success over the last decade. ML is the utmost well-known subset of AI, with applications in a variety of fields including natural language processing (NLP), computer graphics, speech recognition, computer vision, intelligent control and decision-making. Additionally, ML has the ability to support computer networks also. Some studies looked at how ML could be used to resolve and explain networking issues like resource allocation, security, routing, traffic engineering, etc.

The importance of edge intelligence is also growing rapidly as the requirement for integrated real-time remote services reaches new heights. Customers would like to have applications at their disposal so that they can quickly gain insights and feel secure about their results. With AI-powered capabilities, the data from the IoT devices can be analysed, transformed, visualized and embedded through the entire ecosystem – edge devices, gateways, routers and data centres, in the cloud.

5.2.1   DATA ANALYTICS VS. MACHINE LEARNING

ML at the most basic level takes vast volumes of data and turns it into valuable insights for businesses. This could include streamlining procedures, lowering prices, providing a better customer service or introducing new business models. The thing is all of these advantages can be obtained by using conventional data analytics rather than more complex ML methods in the most cases.

Traditional data analysis excels at providing context for data. You may create reports or models based on what has been in the past or what is currently happening and then apply those lessons to the organization. Data analytics will help you measure and monitor your objectives, make better decisions and track your progress over time.

5.2.2   SO WHEN IS MACHINE LEARNING VALUABLE?

Classic data analytics models are often static and ineffective in dealing with rapidly shifting unstructured and dynamic data. Finding relations between thousands of sensor elements and external dynamics that generate large number of data points is frequently critical in IoT environment. The conventional data analysis process requires building a model based on historical data to create a correlation between the variables. On the other hand, ML begins with the outcome variables (e.g. energy savings) and then searches for predictor variables and their relations automatically.

Human beings require learning activities with the purpose of comprehending and identifying various elements such as a speech, an individual, an entity and others. Acquiring knowledge by generalization, in which we typically construct models from training samples to identify new trends and scenarios, is generally distinguished from learning by memorization. It is simple for machines to manage an enormous amount of data; however, it is more difficult to create a good model that can efficiently recognize new objects in a new test. ML procedures are an attempt to comprehend and replicate this learning ability in a machine.

5.2.3   TYPES OF MACHINE LEARNING

ML techniques are mainly categorized into following four categories:

a) **Supervised Learning:** It is a method for generating rules without human intervention from database samples that have already been administered and validated. The principal goal is to arrange the future data using a classification model that has already been driven by these samples. The preferred output labels, on the other hand, are known from the start. As a result, in the training process, where the task is to construct a model by analysing previously known parameters, human interaction (supervisor) is critical.

The aim of creating a decision-making model is to predict the values of the output variable for each observation based on the values of the other input variables. There are two cases when we are dealing with a decision model: the explained variable in a problem of division between two or more classes is called as nominal variable, each of whose modality corresponds to one of the potential classes. The explained variable in a regression problem is called as quantitative variable. Likewise, the explained variable in a structured prediction problem receives values from a structured data domain.

In supervised learning, the algorithm's robustness is determined by the accuracy of its preparation. Data extraction is predictive when an algorithm learns supervised content and creates an internal model that can be reused to identify new volumes of data. Further, there are two types of algorithms for supervised learning:

(i) **Classification:** When the output or target variable is a category, such as 'black' or 'white' or 'trustworthy' and 'un-trustworthy'.

(ii) **Regression:** When the target variable is a value, such as 'sales' or 'weight'

Various steps included in supervised learning are shown in Figure 5.1.

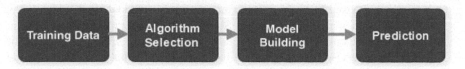

Figure 5.1 Steps in supervised learning

b) **Unsupervised Learning:** It is one of the ML techniques which works with unlabelled heterogeneous data. It splits the given data set into subgroups based on heterogeneity. Within a homogeneous group, the data that is considered to be the most similar is linked. Dissimilar records, on the other hand, are grouped together in other categories. In general, the aim is to enable the extraction of structured information from this data.

The data in this learning class is not labelled, so the learning procedure must find common features among its input data on its own. ML approaches that promote unsupervised learning are particularly valuable as unlabelled data is more plentiful as compared to labelled data. The most significant distinction between supervised and unsupervised learning is that the latter does not necessitate human involvement. Data extraction is descriptive since the algorithm can figure out how to distinguish between artefacts on its own by searching for similarities. Unsupervised learning can be further classified into two categories:

  (i) **Clustering:** A clustering problem is one in which you want to determine the data's underlying relationships, such as grouping customers based on their shopping habits.
  (ii) **Association:** In this kind of unsupervised learning problem, one learns about the rules which define the major portion of the data.

Unsupervised learning is summarized in Figure 5.2.

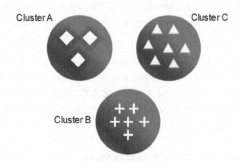

Figure 5.2 Clustering in unsupervised learning

c) **Semi-supervised Learning:** The data set must be hand labelled, which is the most fundamental drawback of any Supervised Learning algorithm. This is an extremely expensive method, especially when working with large amounts of data. Unsupervised learning's most basic drawback is that its implementation range is small. The principle of semi-supervised learning was developed to address these drawbacks. The algorithm is trained on a mixture of labelled and unlabelled data in this method of learning. This mixture would usually contain a lesser volume of labelled data compared to the large volume of unlabelled data.

The basic technique entails the programmer clustering related data using an unsupervised learning algorithm before labelling the remaining unlabelled data with the existing labelled data. The standard use cases for this form of algorithm all have one thing in common: acquiring unlabelled data is relatively inexpensive, whereas labelling the same data is extremely costly. The resulting classifying function in the case of a semi-supervised classifier is restricted to the labels class given in the set of pre-classified input instances. However, in the case of semi-supervised clustering, on the other hand, the function of the resulting classifier is free to add new labels or remove them if the spatial structure of the input instances is compatible.

d) **Reinforcement Learning:** It is a form of ML technique that learns what needs to be done based on previous experiences so as to obtain the best solution. Reinforcement learning is described as the learning through communication with the environment and observation of the results of a specific behaviour. It enables machines to automatically evaluate the optimal behaviour in a given situation with the intention to optimize their productivity. To learn how the machines must behave, a simple return of the results is needed.

Reinforcement learning is an emerging field of machine learning that involves agents (software applications) that take actions in order to get the maximum reward. This technique is mainly based on a) an agent, which is committed to an action in its present state; b) environment, which provides inputs based on the actions taken, c) Reward, which is an incentive provided by the environment; d) current state provided by the environment and e) action that an agent can take. The process flow of the reinforcement learning is shown in Figure 5.3.

The above-discussed ML techniques are summarized in Table 5.1 along with the type of input data they deal with and the purpose of using these algorithms.

Next, some of the common uses of these ML techniques are weather forecasting, sales prediction, gaming industry, healthcare, social network, finance, etc. These applications are illustrated in Figure 5.4.

5.2.4 MODEL PERFORMANCE EVALUATION

The main objective of every ML technique is to use factual inputs to construct a model which works better in practical circumstances and can be evaluated

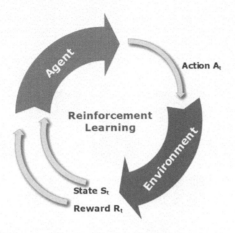

Figure 5.3   Process flow of reinforcement learning

quantitatively and reproducibly. Valuation of mathematical models is a subfield in and of itself, but we'll go over the fundamentals that apply to nearly all the ML algorithms that will come across.

a) **Confusion Matrix:** In classification models, to evaluate the performance, an $n \times n$ matrix is used where n is the number of target categories or classes. This

Table 5.1
Classification of Machine Learning Techniques

ML Technique	Input Data	Purpose
Supervised Learning	Labelled data	Making predictions by learning parameters
Unsupervised Learning	Unlabelled data	Displaying data distribution without making a distinction between the observed and unobserved data variables, as well as the variables that will be expected
Semi-Supervised Learning	Combination of labelled data and unlabelled data	For providing trends and distribution along with making decisions
Reinforcement Learning	Rewards	Learning with experience-driven process and decision-making through the use of incentives.

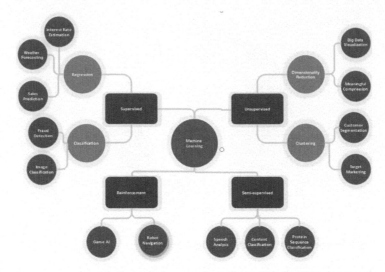

Figure 5.4 Some common examples where machine learning algorithms can be used.

$n \times n$ matrix is also known as confusion matrix. It is used for comparing the actual values with predicted values. This comparison provides an estimation on model's classification power and also tells about the errors the model is making.

In case of a binary classifier (where there are only two categories to predict), the target variable can have either a positive value or a negative value. The columns of the confusion matrix as shown in Figure 5.5 denote original values (actual values) and rows denote expected values (predicted values) of the target variable. Based on the values of the target variable (either positive or negative), we can have the following cases:

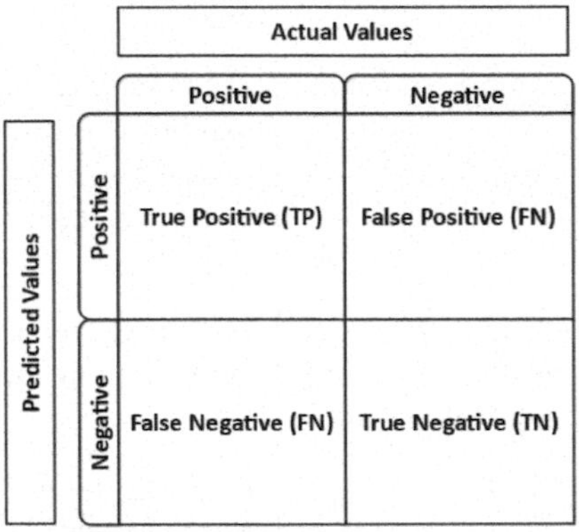

		Actual Values	
		Positive	Negative
Predicted Values	Positive	True Positive (TP)	False Positive (FN)
	Negative	False Negative (FN)	True Negative (TN)

Figure 5.5 Confusion Matrix

(i) If the target variable's predicted value matches the actual value, then it can be *true positive (TP)* (if the target variable's original value is positive and the model is also predicted as positive) or *true negative (TN)* (if the target variable's original value is negative and the model is also predicted as negative).

(ii) If the predicted value of the target variable does not match with the actual value, then it can be *false positive (FP)* (if the target variable's real value is negative; however, the value predicted by the model is positive also known as *Type 1 error*) or *false negative (FN)* (if the target variable's real value is positive; however, the value predicted by the model is negative also known as *Type 2 error*).

Let's consider an example to understand the confusion matrix. Let's presume the objective is to calculate the number of individuals who are sick with an infectious virus until they exhibit the signs, and separate them from the stable population. The target variable can have the values 1 and 0 where 1 represents the infected population and 0 represents the stable population.

Let's assume that a model was built on a data set with 1000 patients, and it is shown in Figure 5.6. The predictions for the target variable were as follows:

Patient ID	Actual	Predicted	Performance
1	1	1	TP
2	0	1	FP
3	0	0	TN
4	1	0	FN
		.	
		.	
1000	0	0	TN

Figure 5.6   An example table that shows model performance in terms of TP, TN, FP and FN for a data set with 1000 observations

Out of 1000 observations, $TP = 50$, $TN = 910$, $FP = 10$ and $FN = 30$. The accuracy of a model is computed using the following formula:

$$Accuracy = \frac{TP + TN}{(TN + TP + FN + FP)}$$

In the above case,

$$Accuracy = \frac{50 + 910}{910 + 50 + 30 + 10} = 0.96$$

The above percentage states that the model is able to predict infected patients 96% of the time. However, by looking at the value of TN, the model, in reality, is predicting patients who will not get infected with the accuracy of 96%. The main objective is to calculate the patients who will get infected (TP); to stop the virus from spreading or to check the reliability of the model, we should calculate the infected patients out of the predicted cases. Hence, additional metrics are required to represent model performance.

b) **Positive predictive value (PPV) and negative predictive value (NPV)**: Positive predictive value or precision is the probability that subjects with a positive screening test truly have the disease. This gives an idea about the reliability of the model. When accessing the achievability or the success of a screening program, positive and negative predictive values should always be taken into consideration. These are also calculated from the same $n \times n$ contingency table; however, the perspective is entirely different.

$$PPV = \frac{TP}{TP + FP}$$

Taking the above example,

$$PPV = \frac{50}{50 + 10} = 0.83$$

This means 83% of the total positives predicted by the model were actually positive. Negative predictive value is the probability that patients with negative screening results genuinely are not infected.

$$NPV = \frac{TN}{TN + FN}$$

$$NPV = \frac{910}{910 + 30} = 0.96$$

PPV and NPV should definitely be considered while assessing the success or practicality of a program. Both the values can be calculated by using the same confusion matrix.

c) **Sensitivity vs. specificity**: Sensitivity and specificity play an important role in performance validation of ML or mathematical model. These are used to determine whether a model is working as required or not. As a result, it is vital to consider what both of these quantities teach us about what a learned model can and cannot do. Sensitivity is the likelihood that a positive outcome will arise if the sample is still positive. In other words, it is the percentage of true positives. For example, 70% sensitivity implies 70% of the patients who are suffering from the target illness will test positive. Sensitivity or the true positive rate is also known as the strike rate or more commonly recall and equal to $1 - FNR$. In mathematical terms,

$$Sensitivity = \frac{TP}{(TP + FN)}$$

Specificity is the likelihood of a negative outcome given a negative sample. It is also known as the true negative rate and is calculated as the percentage of true negatives. For example, 70% specificity implies 70% of the patients who are not suffering from the target illness will test negative. It corresponds to 1 − FPR. In mathematical terms,

$$Specificity = \frac{TN}{(TN + FP)}$$

d) **The receiver operator curve (ROC) and area under the curve (AUC):** The ROC is a standard metric for evaluating the output of statistical models. The ROC can be represented by a numeric value ranging from 0 to 1. It represents the estimated area under the ROC curve. This curve is a two-dimensional map that shows the comparison between the false-positive rate and the true-positive rate. A test's effectiveness is determined by four values: true negative rate, true-positive rate (TPR), false-negative rate and false-positive rate (FPR). TP and TN are right test responses; on the other hand, FP and false-negative FN are erroneous solutions. The aforementioned values can be further broken down into two categories: sensitivity and specificity which have been discussed above. Therefore, now let's calculate ROC using them.

In an ideal situation, a test will have high sensitivity as well as a high specificity. However, there is a trade-off; prioritizing one always means sacrificing the other. If we adjust the threshold low enough, then it yields a high TPR (high sensitivity) but also a high FPR (low specificity). Adjusting the threshold too high, on the other hand, would result in a low TPR (low sensitivity) and also low FPR (high specificity).

The ROC and AUC metrics are used to classify the majority of the categorization tasks that many statistical models seek to perform; does this individual have the disease or not? In an ideal scenario, a test will have high sensitivity and specificity, and the AUC score is equal to 1. In aforementioned curves, FPR lies on the x-axis and TPR lies on the y-axis. In an ideal condition, the FPR should be as low as possible for the model to work at its best. One more way of interpreting AUC is by percentage, i.e. a percentage that the model is able to distinguish goods from bads. For example, a 0.83 ROC score denotes that the model has 83% possibility to successfully identify whether a case is true or false.

There are a few other metrics also for estimating ML model performance. Some of these performance metrics are logarithmic loss, F1-score, mean absolute error, mean squared error, etc.

5.3 APPLICATION OF IOT AND MACHINE LEARNING IN HEALTHCARE

To better understand the connection between IoT and ML techniques, the IoT-based healthcare system has been considered in this chapter. Various surveys like

[154–156] on IoT and ML in healthcare present a review on various techniques comprising of IoT frameworks and ML algorithms in healthcare department. Healthcare is concerned with the collection, delivery, analysis, storage and retrieval of data related to healthcare for the purposes of disease detection, diagnosis and treatment. The application of healthcare is limited to disease-related data, medical records and the statistical methods used to process such data [157]. Traditional medical practices across the world have invested in improved technologies and computational support for researchers, medical professionals and patients in the last few decades with the aim of delivering accessible, high-quality and streamlined healthcare. Wrist-worn devices can be used for flexible and better monitoring of the patients [158]. Computerized physician order entry (CPOE), for example, has been shown to minimize prescription errors and adverse drug events while unwittingly improving treatment quality. When doctors enter a prescription for a patient, CPOE makes patient details readily available to them. It gives the doctor the information he or she needs about potential adverse reactions based on the patient's past. Furthermore, CPOE enables the practitioner to keep track of the order. This offers a new way for the doctors to spot problems with prescriptions and rewrite them to eliminate errors and correct inaccuracies. ML is a subclass of AI, and it aims to automate complex time-consuming tasks [159]. When dealing with complex statistical analysis, researchers, scientists and medical consultants often turn to ML. Healthcare informatics is the field that combines together clinical data and ML with the aim of detecting trends of interest. Therefore, the purpose of using ML in healthcare is to find trends in data and then learn from them before taking any critical decision.

Innovative methods for capturing diseases such as cancers have emerged as a result of technological advancements in medical imaging. Cancers can now be detected and diagnosed more effectively thanks to these advancements. Minimally invasive surgery, image-driven therapy and accurate monitoring of treatment response have all been made possible by prominent imaging modalities such as computed tomography (CT) ultrasound, and magnetic resonance imaging (MRI). Anatomical data on the size, shape and position of tumours and growths is now possible thanks to these technologies.

Popular imaging techniques, for instance, ultrasound, MRI and CT scan have made successful implementation of medical procedures such as image-guided therapy, minimally invasive surgery and precise evaluation of treatment reaction. These developments also allowed the collection of anatomical data on the size, form and location of tumours. Data analysis methods are widely classified as descriptive, exploratory, inferential, predictive and causal. An exploratory analysis process establishes correlations among the features in a data set, while a descriptive analysis summarizes the data with no explanation.

ML is the method of learning a strong enough mathematical model to forecast results or categories of findings in future data using observed data. Supervised machine learning systems, in particular, train a model using observations on specimens where the category or expected value of the target is already known. The resulting model is usually applied to new samples to categorize or forecast values of the outcome for previously unseen experiments, and its accuracy is tested by comparing expected values to real values for a series of test samples. As a result, ML 'exists' in the field of algorithmic simulation and can be assessed as such. Regression models created using machine learning techniques cannot and should not be tested using data modelling principles [160]. This would result in inaccurate assessments of a model's results for its intended task, ultimately leading to incorrect perception of the model's production by users.

Electronic health records (EHRs) open the gates to a large variety and quantity of variables, allowing high-quality classification and prediction [161], while ML provides methods for dealing with the large numbers of high-dimensional data which is common in a healthcare environment. Additionally, the implementation of ML techniques to EHR data processing is at the forefront of the present-day clinical informatics [156], accelerating advancements in both medicine's research and practice.

IoT-Based healthcare platforms can be used for monitoring patients remotely [162]. This includes real-time data analysis to manage monitoring of data from various resources such as sensors, as well as the interpretation of continuous data for use in intensive care units (ICU). Similarly, considerable research effort has been directed over the last two decades towards the monitoring and classification of human body movements and patterns from the data from body-wearable sensors.

Measures for analysing sensors' data are starting to play a vital role in high-level epidemiological studies in this field, as self-reported measures are indicated to be inaccurate indicators for activity profiling. Computer-aided diagnosis (CAD) and its related methods have been critical in realizing ML's potential. In the field of cancer science, there are numerous CAD methods. This is due to the large amount of data that can be used to create such tools. However, there is a need for efficient data and information integration from multiple data sources.

A range of health threats have already been characterized and predicted using ML methods. Recent research in our community showed that the performance of a penalty-based logistic regression surpasses the performance of a simplified step-wise logistic regression in segmenting patients suffering from undetected peripheral artery disease and estimating the risk of mortality. This comparison was done on the basis of calibration, precision and net reclassification [163].

These kind of predictive models have been applied in medical practice which ensures highly effective and higher quality treatment. When Kaiser Permanente implemented a statistical approach to stratify newborns' danger of sepsis, it reduced the antibiotic recommendations by 33%–60% [164]. A recent work to acquire heart and respiratory rate comparison ranges from EHR data culminated in a reduction in heart rate alarms in a paediatric intensive care unit following the introduction of the learned ranges in unit monitors, minimizing warning fatigue.

ML techniques are being used in hospital and clinic administration for optimizing patient outcomes and streamline processes. To guide hospital staffing decisions, models are built to estimate the need for elective surgery patient volume [165] and emergency department beds [166]. The Veterans Health Administration's Clinical Data Warehouse contains medical data for more than 20 million people. It was utilized to build models for hospitalization risk and mortality of particular patients with 0.81 to 0.87 AUC values [167].

IoT devices with the help of thermal sensors can be used to detect people having high fever in crowded places [168]. Similarly, with the appropriate integration of networks, medical machines and appliances, healthcare treatment system and services, a infrastructure can be built to address patients with medical conditions [169].

General steps involved with ML and IoT can be summarized as follows:

1. The addition of machine sensors helps measure discrete variables such as noise, vibration, heat and temperature. The data is then moved to the cloud for review and analysis.

2. ML now enters the picture; the ML model is hosted on the cloud platform and feeds on incoming data.

3. The ML model divides the data into two categories: training and verification.

4. To generate a hypothesis, the model examines hundreds of thousands of data sets for anomalies, associations and predictions.

5. The hypothesis must be tested and confirmed after it has been established.

6. A model is released as an executable endpoint once it has been validated. The live streaming data can then be fed into the trained model, which can then make an inference about the machinery's status/health based on what it has been trained on and to search for.

5.3.1   CASE STUDY 1

The healthcare industry may be further subdivided into physical and mental health services. The healthcare sector has shifted from physical to mental healthcare over the last decade. Alzheimer's syndrome is one of the most common mental health disorders among the elderly population. The Alzheimer's Association survey (2018) backs this up. For patients suffering from Alzheimer's, ML-based solution can be implemented for distinguishing between Alzheimer's patients and patients with mild mental illness. For automatically diagnosing Alzheimer's syndrome, a multi-template ML system can be implemented. A model can be built with the help of feature selection and SVM algorithms. An experiment was conducted on 12 Alzheimer's affected women and 12 women with no health issues. The calculations indicated that better classification accuracy can be achieved by making use of SVM for feature selection. Similarly, an IoT-Based cloud healthcare mechanism can be implemented to predict severe illness. A better solution to detect an illness in a patient's body would be to use a multi-layered model.

Below is an example to detect Alzheimer's disease in a three-level architecture:

1. The first level involves determining whether or not the person under supervision is an Alzheimer's patient. Recurrent neural network (RNN), a common deep learning approach, is used for this purpose. RNN is made up of many computing layers that have an agenda to think about data representations by

abstraction. To forecast Alzheimer's patients, the sensory system's input data is fed into the RNN model.

2. At the second level, a collaborative method for monitoring Alzheimer's patient's abnormality is planned during this process to minimize the count of incorrect detections generated by the model. It can be done by analysing patient's verbal and visual actions. If the output of the collective values from these analyses is greater than the recommended trigger value, then the patient requires assistance.

3. The last level of the model includes making use of IoT devices. This step is required to provide appropriate help to the patient with positive Alzheimer's. The assistance is provided based on the trigger produced in level two.

The three-level process explained above is shown in Figure 5.7.

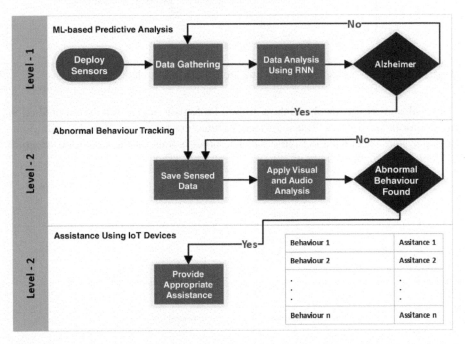

Figure 5.7   IoT- and machine learning–based framework to detect Alzheimer's and provide assistance to the patients

5.3.2   CASE STUDY 2

The suggested ML and IoT-Based health monitoring model is built on a three-tier system that can store and process massive amounts of data from wearable sensors. Tier 1 collects data from IoT wearable sensor systems. Tier 2 stores the massive amount of raw data in the cloud using Apache HBase sent by the several IoT sensors.

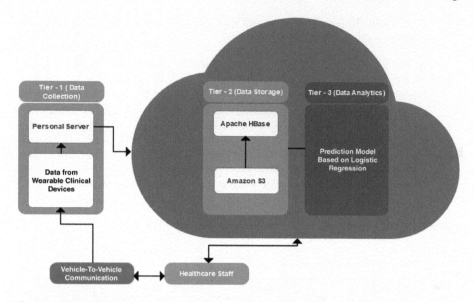

Figure 5.8   IoT- and ML-based healthcare framework to detect heart disease

Tier 3 also employs Apache Mahout to build a logistic regression–based prediction model for heart diseases. The suggested architecture for an IoT-Based health monitoring system is depicted in Figure 5.8. The process flow for the suggested structure is depicted in Figure 5.9

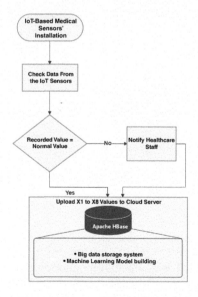

Figure 5.9   IoT- and ML-based healthcare data flow process

1. **Data Collection:** The intended IoT- and ML-based health management architecture is divided into three sections: data collection, data storage and data analytics. The data collection block is used to collect physiological data from individuals via wearable IoT sensor devices. IoT wearable sensors connected to the human body continuously gather health data from the patient. When an individual's clinical measure approaches its threshold value, the machines give a warning massage with the clinical value to the healthcare staff and the treatment owners.

   The warning notifications and therapeutic values are continuously compiled and recorded in the database. The suggested mechanism makes use of 5G cell networks to migrate health data into a clinical archive, allowing for the appropriate response in any kind of emergency situation. The proposed IoT-Based health management system transfers clinical data from a local disk to a cloud network using the 's3cmd' process.

2. **Data Storage:** In general, IoT devices are designed to transmit clinical data in real time. Conventional data collection methods and strategies struggle to store and handle such massive amounts of data. The proposed architecture stores clinical data in a distributed way using big data technology. Apache HBase is an essential component of distributed data management. Physical devices and personal computers are insufficient for storing the massive amounts of data provided by IoT wearable devices. The proposed IoT-Based health monitoring framework addresses the issue with the use of cloud computing technology for scalability and elasticity.

   To obtain virtual machines with Apache HBase database access, an Amazon account is built. Health-related data obtained from the patient's body is initially moved to the Amazon easy storage facility S3 using the 's3cmd utility' tool. As a result, when an individual's clinical measure reaches the usual value, the IoT devices transfer the clinical measurements to Amazon S3. In comparison with Amazon S3, Apache HBase offers a distributed modular data management system. As a result, clinical data is moved from Amazon S3 to Apache HBase. The suggested health management system transfers clinical data from Amazon S3 to Apache HBase using Apache Pig.

   Apache Pig is commonly used for extracting, loading and transforming massive amounts of semi-structured, unstructured and structured data. PigLatin is a language that is used in Apache Pig to execute data transformations. Wearable IoT sensors are attached to the human body to capture physiological data. These instruments provide a vast amount of data that cannot be contained in conventional databases. As a result, the Hadoop distributed file system is used to store vast amounts of data in a scalable fashion.

3. **Data Analytics:** This block is expected to construct the prediction model by applying logistic regression. The suggested architecture implements logistic regression technique for estimating the coefficient value between a dependent variable and one or more independent variables using Apache Mahout-based

machine learning libraries. Logistic regression functions similarly to linear regression, in addition to the dependent variable.

In linear regression, the dependent variable Y and the independent variable X contain numeric values; however on the other hand, in logistic regression, the independent variable X may also contain categorical values. The dependent variable Y is coded as 1 in most instances and 0 in others. Multiple logistic regression is described as follows:

$$logit(p) = b0 + b1X1 + b2X2 + ... + bkXk$$

where the probability of the inclusion of the dependent variable is denoted by p (heart disease 0 or 1), coefficients are denoted by b, Xi stands for independent variables, i denotes the number of therapeutic parameters, $X1$ = respiratory rate (RP), $X2$ = heart rate (HR), $X3$ = blood pressure-systolic range (BP-SR), $X4$ = blood pressure-diastolic range (BP-DR), $X5$ = body temperature (BT), $X6$ = blood sugar – fasting (BS-F) and $X7$ = blood sugar – post meal (BS-PM).

This health surveillance architecture employs logistic regression to build a prediction model for the early detection of heart diseases. In cloud computing, Apache Mahout is used in conjunction with the Elastic MapReduce (EMR) paradigm to create prediction models. Once the clinical data is stored in Apache HBase, the Mahout-based logistic regression develops a predictive model dependent on the previous clinical records.

As a constantly emerging area, machine learning has a wide variety of possible uses in the healthcare discipline, which may include secondary areas such as staff control, insurance plans, regulatory affairs, etc. Among many applications of machine learning in healthcare, one use of it is in medical images such as magnetic resonance imaging (MRI), computerized axial tomography (CAT) scans, ultrasound imaging and positron emission tomography (PET) scans. The end product of these imaging modalities is a sequence or series of photographs that must be interpreted and diagnosed by a radiologist. ML techniques are increasingly improving in their ability to forecast and locate photographs that may signify a disease state or serious problem.

Many healthcare practitioners agree that the drive towards electronic medical records (EMR) in many countries is sluggish, boring and, in many cases, totally botched. This will also result in patients receiving significantly poorer healthcare. The number of physical patient records and paperwork that still remain in many hospitals and clinics is one of the biggest challenges. Different formatting, handwritten note and a plethora of missing or non-centralized data have made the transition to electronic medical records comparatively less efficient.

Another application of machine learning in the healthcare department incorporates the use of human genetics to forecast illness and identify disease causes. With the arrival of next-generation sequencing (NGS) techniques and the abundance of genetic data, including vast data sets of population-wide genetic information, the effort to discern useful information about how human health condition is affected by genetics is now at the forefront of many research endeavours. Understanding how complex disorders manifest and how evolution can improve or reduce an individual's risk can help with pre-emptive healthcare. It can give doctors more insight on how to customize a patient's treatment plan to eliminate the chance of developing more complicated diseases.

5.3.3 KEY CHALLENGES AND LIMITATIONS

As discussed earlier, the IoT can be one of the greatest benefits to healthcare; however, there are numerous challenges that need to be addressed. Apart from the risk of failure, one of the major challenge is security and privacy of the data. Patients' data should be secure and not leaked in any circumstances. We need a secure technique for authentication and transmission of data from one device to another [170]. Another challenge is the accuracy of the data. Since a large amount of data needs to be processed at a real-time basis, there is a possibility of error while handling the data. Additionally, scalability and interoperability issues may occur while working on a large network [171].

6 Medical IoT: Opportunities, Issues in Security and Privacy - A Comprehensive Review

Deepa Krishnan and Swapnil Singh

CONTENTS

6.1 INTRODUCTION

We are witnessing a world where a pandemic has severely limited the medical fraternity in operating at their full potential because disease management has to be administered remotely many a times. This introduces the need for increased technical support for the healthcare sector. Automating the diagnostic process can help reduce the load on hospitals and doctors and deliver timely medical care to the needy across the globe. With its far-reaching potential, the Internet of Things (IoT) is such a method of automation that can remarkably impact the healthcare industry. Medical

DOI: 10.1201/9781003239895-6

IoT inherently consists of sensors that can record various body vitals like glucose level, blood pressure, pulse rate, heart rate, etc., and can be sent to cloud servers where data analytics and machine learning algorithms can deliver valuable insights.

As stated earlier, the use of IoT has revolutionized the medical sector. Healthcare systems use IoT devices to create an infrastructure that monitors health parameters and automatically acts whenever medical intervention is required [172]. The IoT-based medical devices may be more economically beneficial in the long run. However, that is not the only reason for the increased adoption of IoT in the healthcare sector. The shortage of paramedics and doctors is likely to boost the adoption of IoT devices in the medical sector. It is expected that the USA alone will face a shortage of 125000 physicians by 2025, and this shortage is likely to be greater in Asia and Africa. According to BI Intelligence, around 161 million medical IoT devices have been in use since 2020; the trends of the expected number of Health IoT devices installed globally are shown in Figure 6.1 [173]. As seen in Figure 6.2, the medical IoT market is expected to grow to 135.87 billion dollars by the year 2025 [174]; IoT devices can be particularly useful where social distancing norms are being enforced to control the COVID-19 pandemic.

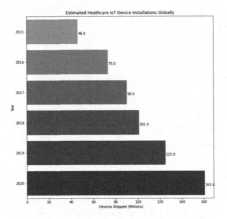

Figure 6.1   Expected healthcare IoT device installations globally [173]

With the help of IoT, we can set up better and more efficient remote health-monitoring systems; REMOA is one such project that targets home solutions for the health monitoring of patients with chronic illnesses. This system includes strategies and protocols for data transfer between different sensing devices like movement sensors and blood pressure monitors. All sensors are connected wirelessly to each other and the central monitor. The monitor is responsible for accommodating, aggregating and comparing the collected information against series. When the limit is crossed, it can raise the alarm and trigger the health workers to react promptly to the health-related event [172].

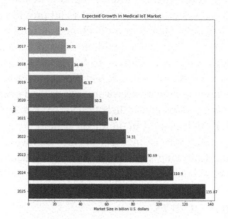

Figure 6.2   Expected growth in medical IoT market [174]

According to WHO, 17.9 million people die of cardiovascular disease every year. Four out of five patients suffering from heart diseases die due to heart attacks and strokes. One-third of such deaths are premature in people under the age of 70. Regular monitoring and check-ups could reduce the risk of such diseases and help prevent strokes and heart attacks. However, regular monitoring inconveniences the patients greatly and might not even yield the data useful for medical prognosis or diagnosis. IoT-Based monitoring devices mitigate these inconveniences and can be more efficient and reliable. Intelligent monitoring solutions can trigger emergency medical intervention when body vitals show anomalies. Smart health motoring is an amalgamation of intelligent computing in addition to remote health monitoring with IoT. The body sensor network constitutes various wearable or implantable devices like cardioverter–defibrillator and pacemakers, which can sense and monitor blood pressure, heart rate and other such vitals of the body. These devices stack the data in a clinical data set, which can later be referred [175].

IoT is vigorously promoted in healthcare by all leading global healthcare institutions. Microsoft developed intelligent systems to formulate a structure to capture health data from IoT devices, thus ensuring the required connectivity. Intel aims to bring healthcare any time and anywhere. It emphasizes synchronizing health data streaming and communication systems in real time to lower the cycle time and the first-time quality of many existing medial work flow environments. In collaboration with various well-known firms, IBM has developed IoT devices for a series of healthcare solutions like health analytics of healthcare data, data governance of healthcare data and connected home health. Apple came up with the Apple Watch to monitor your blood oxygen levels, heart rate and blood pressure. The Memorial Hermann healthcare system entirely relies on Apple's solution for providing connection and efficient healthcare, giving secure access, physician gains and better care. Cisco is working with various health organizations to build a health-grade network architecture, deploy converged system-based networks and provide algorithms to handle substantial incoming IoT data. Qualcomm developed an integrated solution that can capture and deliver real-time data from health devices to databases and portals. The Indian Government took various initiatives to boost the use of IoT in the medical sector. Countries like the USA, Australia, Japan, France, Germany, China and Korea have already taken various healthcare sector initiatives, and even the Indian Government has also started taking steps in this direction [176]. We can see a growing influx of a wide variety of IoT devices used in the medical field.

There are different categories of medical IoT devices which are used in today's connected world. In the following section, we have described some important categories of IoT devices based on their utility.

6.1.1 WEARABLE IOT DEVICES

We can categorize IoT devices as per their application as i) IoT for toddlers, ii) IoT for kids, iii) IoT for chronic care, iv) IoT for motion detection and body motion reconstruction, v) IoT for personal emergency response systems, vi) IoT for surgery guidance and vii) IoT in mobility aids. Mimo, an example of IoT for toddlers, is a resting device built to monitor respiration, sleeping position and body temperature; it then collects the data and sends it to the working parents. Another such example is Milk Nanny; this device makes warm baby milk using milk powder, all of this with a press of a button on the phone. TempTraq is a Bluetooth patch that tracks the baby's temperature and sends the data to the caretaker's mobile phone. Smart diapers are another example of an IoT device for toddlers, which is a thin sensor placed in the diaper which informs the caretaker that it is the time to change the diaper [177].

iSwimband is an IoT device for kids; it is a Bluetooth-connected device; if the device is submerged for a user-defined time, it alerts the connected iOS device. Sleep monitoring systems are also an excellent example of the use of IoT devices for kids. These systems track the natural sleeping environment, body parameters like temperature, blood pressure and movement while sleeping. IoT devices are also being used for chronic care; these can be implants or wearable devices. Wearable devices include temperature sensors and CO sensors to prevent breathing. [177]

Wearable motion trackers are used to monitor body motion; the sensor is placed at rotational angles and lower extremity joints. The data collected from these sensors can be used for tumour detection. This system is activated in the ICU when we need to track the activities of the patient. Certain devices are used for personal emergency response. Blood pressure measurement sensors are one such example of these devices. Google glasses are used for a higher percentage of success in surgeries; Google glasses help doctors to confirm their decision during surgery. Pathfinder wheelchairs and stretchers are very useful as mobility aids; these are IoT devices for finding a path. Gemalto has developed an automatic pill dispenser consisting of IoT, mobile phones and wireless M2M. The pillbox is wirelessly connected to the patient, doctor, family member and medical alert monitoring centre. [177]

6.1.2 IMPLANTABLE MEDICAL DEVICES

Besides the patient monitoring devices, many IoT devices embedded in the human body could track and report body parameters. The recent advances in nanocircuits and manufacturing materials for in-body devices have propelled the growth and popularity of implantable devices. Implantable devices are placed in the human body through a medical procedure and left in the body. Some of these are even capable of regulating and alter vital statistics of the human body. For instance, some examples are cardiac pacemakers, coronary stents and implantable insulin pumps, to name a few. Cardiac pacemakers are used in patients whose heart rhythm is prone to be very high or too low or impeded due to any heart trauma [178]. Another popular device is an insulin pump surgically inserted into the abdominal tissue and releases basal insulin via a catheter [179]. It is highly efficient than conventional wearable insulin because it is delivered to the peritoneal cavity and released in a controlled way to the body. The cardiac stents with a vast user base worldwide are popular among these implantable devices. They are used to improve the blood flow in blocked coronary arteries.

6.1.3 STATIONARY MEDICAL IOT DEVICES

Stationary devices are used to measure physiological parameters, and the most commonly used are nuclear imaging devices, X-ray and mammography devices, ultrasound machines, CT and MRI scanners. These are comparatively costly and sophisticated devices that transmit diagnostic images wirelessly to physicians and are generally used by hospitals and diagnostics centres. These images are collected and integrated into the patient's electronic health record (EHR). Stationary medical devices help in timely diagnosis and are integrated with other knowledge management systems; this aids in quick and efficient decision-making. Most IoT devices use Wi-Fi, Bluetooth and Zigbee technology to communicate with peer devices and the server [180]. Besides, near field communication (NFC) has also observed that cellular and satellite communication have also been used for end-to-end connectivity of remote patients with healthcare infrastructure. The use of innovative technology in healthcare has been increasing in recent years, and this is further accelerated with the challenges thrown by the COVID-19 pandemic. The easiness with which consumers embraced smart healthcare will propel its usage further in the coming years.

6.2 PRIVACY AND SECURITY ISSUES IN MEDICAL IOT

We have discussed the potential applications of IoT in the medical sector in Section 6.1. As stated in the above section, IoT has several advantages, like being cost-friendly and remote monitoring. Along with these advantages, we have several problems and issues, raising concerns for using IoT in the medical sector. IoT devices in the medical field are deployed with minimal security features and are prone to attacks like denial of power attacks, eavesdropping, tampering parameter configurations, hijacking, device cloning, denial of service (DoS) and tampering messages [181].

Security attacks in IoT devices tend to cause damage, disruption, misdirection, misuse, malfunction or unauthorized access to the device [182].

It is indicative in Figure 6.3 that 41% of the threats for IoT devices in healthcare are of exploit type, including zero-day, network scan, SQL injection, remote code execution, buffer overload, command injection and others; 33% of the threats are due to malware, including botnet, backdoor trojan, ransomware and worm, whereas the rest 26% is due to user practices like line passwords, phishing and cryptojacking. As we observe, there are multiple threats to the security and the privacy of IoT devices in medical care and the patient; therefore, it is the need of the hour to identify these threats and provide solutions to tackle them. It is observed that device manufacturers ignore security aspects while producing IoT products and give more importance to the functionality of devices. One such example is that the IoT-Based glucose monitoring and insulin delivery system frequently launches various security and privacy attacks.

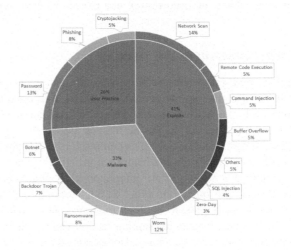

Figure 6.3   Frequently occurring cyberattacks [183]

6.2.1   SECURITY ISSUES IN MEDICAL IOT

The challenges posed by medical IoT devices, unlike other IoT installations, are multi-fold. The consequences are more significant as they can directly affect the health and life of users. In this section, the major categories of security attacks are described as follows:

6.2.1.1   Data Level

Security of medical data concerning confidentiality, integrity and availability is very critical. The different categories of security attacks for medical data are as follows:

a) **Data Leakage:** Collecting and storing a patient's medical records must be done completely and ethically following the previously set norms. In case of such a data breach, cybercriminals can access it, and the data can be sold in illegal markets like the dark web. This would be a violation of privacy regulation and cause possible reputational damage and financial risks. [184]. If the data for a political leader or an essential personality leaks similarly, this data can physically harm that person or even kill the person. The data's confidentiality needs to be preserved so that medical information cannot be leaked to an adversary. Eavesdropping is an attack where the intruder just enters the network and listens to the data being transmitted. Eavesdropping is also known as snooping or sniffing attacks [185]. It is difficult to detect this attack because it does not create any abnormalities in the network. Security vulnerabilities in camera-attached gadgets can raise unwanted surveillance in home environments. Another such passive attack is a traffic analysis attack; the attacker can learn from the data being transferred in the network. If the information is encoded, then the knowledge is indirectly available for the user; the attack aims to understand the communication between the parties. Another such attack is a man-in-the-middle attack, like eavesdropping, but here the intruder can interfere with the connection and compromise the data being transferred. The compromise can be made by modifying, deleting or updating the message.

b) **Deception of Data:** The data collected by the IoT sensors is sent to the data warehouses using broadcasting via the internet. This broadcast characteristic is exploited, and the data being transmitted is tampered. This tampering of data can cause life-threatening risks for patients in critical conditions. Even after the data reaches the data warehouses, the data can still tamper. Tampering of data at the data warehouse level can change the medical history of the patient. IoT medical devices work in a trust-less environment; they are subjected to multiple attacks, as stated earlier, which target the device's integrity and the data collected. Spoofing attacks are the main ways of tampering with the network as well as the data. The attacker fakes the sending address to enter the network. Piggybacking and mimicking are ways to execute such attacks [185, 186]. A way to tamper with the transmission data is to perform a data collision attack. Here collision is performed on purpose by instigating a sensor node to transmit the data at the same time when another node is doing it; this leads to data collision, due to which the header of the data gets changed; when this data reaches the receiving end, the receiver rejects the data after checking the header. This causes the loss of medical data. A selective forwarding attack is tampering with the data being sent to the server via a sensor. The attacker forwards some data flowing in the network and drops the rest; the damage to the data is severe when tampering is done near the base station.

c) **Unavailability of Data:** The data collected by medical IoT devices needs to be available for relevant users in a time of need. DoS attacks make this data inaccessible for medical professionals in such critical times. This might cause a threat to the life of acute patients. In case of myocardial infarction or a heart attack, the data collected by the sensors raises the alarm for the medical professionals to know about the condition. Still, if a DoS attack occurs, the alert won't be raised, and if the person attending the patient isn't alert enough, then the patient's life is in acute danger [184]. As we have seen, the data needs to be available for the legitimate user without any disruption. Another way of rendering the data to be unavailable to the user is by battery drainage attack. The attacker exploits the resource constraints of the device, hence draining down the battery of the device [185]. Battery drainage attacks take place on Implantable Medical Devices (IMD) [181]. A way to make the data unavailable for the legitimate user is by keeping the network busy for a long time. A way to do so is by a desynchronization attack. The attacker tampers with the message sent by a sensor node and generates many copies with a forged sequence number. This leads the WBAN to an infinite cycle; the sensor keeps sending the same message repeatedly, which leads to wastage of resources and keeps the network jammed. The network can also be delayed by repeating the same message or waiting for a message to be sent. A replay attack does this [187].

6.2.1.2   Sensor Level

There are many security and privacy issues at the sensor level in a three-tier IoT device used for healthcare systems. It has been seen that manufacturers at times overlook the security aspects of the device and focus on its functionality. Also, the sensors need to be compact, lightweight and have fewer communication overheads, due to which existing security mechanisms may not be practical for medical IoT devices [184]. Security attacks at the device level are as follows:

a) **Tampering with Hardware:** IoT devices, especially sensor parts, are small and can be physically stolen, exposing the attacker's security information. A stolen device can also be reprogrammed and redeployed by the attacker to listen to the conversations without being noticed. The device could also collect data and then use it to make another attack [184, 187]. The hardware can be tampered with by device capturing, reverse engineering attacks, tampering, side-channel attacks and invasive hardware attacks [185]. Another way of tampering with sensor nodes is by jamming a node's action. The attacker launches a radio signal frequency of broad area network (BAN); the sensor nodes that come in the range of this signal cannot send or receive data [186].

b) **Localization Problems:** IoT devices are localized in a network. In this network of IoT devices, due to the design of IoT devices used in the medical sector, they can move in and out of the network coverage. Thus, it is a challenge to check these devices' movement and identify whether there is an attempt to intrude the network done by the attacker [184]. There are applications in which the exact location of IoT devices in the human body needs to be detected with sufficient precision and accuracy. The tampering of location information can impede the usability of the devices [188].

c) **Self-Healing:** Self-healing allows devices to continue to render their function correctly even after a compromise. The device needs to detect the attack and deploy the appropriate action to tackle the invasion. These self-healing methods deployed cannot be bulky and oversized. The methods need to be lightweight in terms of computational complexity and network overheads [184].

d) **Over-the-air programming:** Over-the-air programming is the most popular way of updating IoT devices with many sensor nodes. This process can lead to various security concerns. While updating the system, if an intruder sensor node is present in the network, it can listen to the updates and introduce foreign identities [184]. Most of the time, installing updates happens remotely and is not often managed by a security practitioner. Over-the-air updates can lead to the introduction of malware that can compromise the device's functionality [189].

e) **Forward and Backward Compatibility:** Forward compatibility is the characteristic due to which the future messages can't be read by a sensor when it leaves the network. Whereas backward compatibility is the characteristic of the sensor when it just enters the network, the past messages are not read by the sensor. Continuous communication is the key for IoT networks used for healthcare; thus, it can cause serious health-related issues for critical patients if messages aren't read [184].

6.2.1.3   Server Level

The digitized medical records of patients are often stored in servers referred to as electronic medical records (EMRs). The security attacks targeting the servers storing EMRs can compromise the integrity of the data. Some of the potential areas of attacks targeting servers are as follows [184–186, 190]:

a) **Malicious Device:** When infected with malware, the data stored in servers can negatively impact the clinical diagnosis the patient is undergoing. This malicious data can tamper with the trends being observed in the patient's vitals or can even change its treatment.

b) **Intruder User:** Data stored in the personal server needs to be accessed when the patient is in a critical condition. The access of this data needs to be in the right hands. If an intruder gets access to this data, they may alter the available information, leading to life-threatening conditions for the patient. Masquerading attacks are examples of such a threat. In this attack, an illegitimate entity poses an authorized entity to gain more privileges than authorized. The attacker may exploit the acquired permissions to perform malicious activities. An impersonation attack is another such attack. The intruder acts like a legitimate entity in an authentication protocol to access the network's resources. In simple words, the attacker gets to know one or more sensor nodes; it then updates its messages accordingly and sends the message on behalf of that node.

In a Sybil attack, the attacker intruder node represents multiple identities in the network. This creates a problem for a geographical routing protocol, where the location information needs to be interchanged between their neighbours and the nodes. It is challenging to identify Sybil attacks due to their high mobility and unpredictable nature. The hello flood attack tries to change the destination address of the sensors' messages, which is done by fooling the sensors with high-powered radio transmission. Intrusion attacks are carried out on wearable devices.

c) **Malware Attacks:** The attacker can install malicious software in medical IoT devices, which can violate the system's security. This software is then disguised and inserted into an application to destroy data; run intrusive or destructive programs; or compromise the reliability, privacy or accuracy of the system's data, entire operating system or a particular application. Some commonly used malware are viruses, worms, Trojan horses, rootkits or other software-based malicious entities that can infect a system. A wormhole attack is made to damage the network topology. The transferred packet is copied and replayed at another location or within the same network without changing the content. This creates a tunnel between the two attackers, which will be used for data transmission; such attacks are silent and are severely dangerous. Table 6.1 summarizes the different types of malware and the attacks performed by them.

Table 6.1
Types of Malware and Its Attacks [191]

Malware Type	Attacks Performed on
Spyware	Authenticity, confidentiality and integrity of the available resources
Keylogger	Authenticity, confidentiality and integrity of the available resources
Trojan Horse	Availability and confidentiality of system resources
Virus	Availability and integrity of system resources
Worm	Available data or other such network resources
Ransomware	Available system resources
Rootkit	Availability, confidentiality, authenticity or integrity of system resources or available data

d) **DoS Attacks:** The attackers can send a high-energy signal to prevent the wireless network from working correctly, like the jamming attacks in the physical layer. Another way to achieve this is by flooding the resource constraints with many requests and thereby congesting the bandwidth. The additional load on the base station can result in a DoS attack; this is done by initiating signalling attacks on a serving base station by activating more than required state signals for blocking it.

e) **Distributed Denial of Service Attacks:** Distributed denial of service (DDoS) attack is performed with the same motive as a DoS attack to hamper the execution. However, multiple compromised devices target the medical IoT device causing a DoS, causing the system to crash. Another such way is by denying the resources to the authorized user, which is called as resource hacking.

Table 6.2 summarizes the various layers of a network model along with the attacks that are targeted at those layers. It also summarizes how to counter these attacks, the type of the attack, whether it is active or passive the location of the attacker and whether the attack is internal, external or both.

6.2.2 PRIVACY ISSUES IN MEDICAL IOT

The growing availability of IoT devices and medical applications based on data analytics captures, stores and analyses large amounts of private patient data. Along with the security issues faced by medical IoT devices, the growing privacy issues posed by IoT applications in the medical field are equally problematic. Some of the critical problems posed are risks to confidential patient data, leakage of corporate medical data, ownership, accountability of the data and patient location leakage. In the following section, we have given a comprehensive analysis of the various privacy issues of medical IoT.

a) *User Data and Identity:* Medical IoT devices and related facilities collect real-time patient data using various body-embedded and wearable devices. The enormous data generated by connected devices ensures faster and economic healthcare, better patient experience and efficient workflow for healthcare professionals. However, the end-users should be concerned with how the data is handled and stored before getting their private data exposed. More user data is collected by medical service providers, like the type of device, contexts, frequency of measurements, measurement readings of vitals and body parameters, and the history of usage [192]. This can lead to a fully interconnected web of health information onto which advanced mining and statistical analysis can be applied to leverage valuable insights.

b) **Data or Record Linkage:** Medical records of patients are collected and analysed concerning their demographics and behaviour. This can lead to identifying a patient and their other existing diseases uniquely. Data linkage typically involves grouping observations from multiple data sources to identify the individual's data uniquely. Various sensitive information such as mental status,

Table 6.2

Classification of Layer-Based Attacks

Layer	Attack	Type of Attack	Counter measures	Location of Attacker
Physical	Sybil attack	Active	Direct validation	Internal
Physical	Jamming	Active	Channel hopping	Internal
Physical	Interception	Active	Jamming	Internal
Physical	Physical tampering	Active	Regular monitoring	Internal
Physical	Eavesdropping	Passive	Jamming	Internal
Physical	Impersonation	Active	Encrypted communication	Internal
Physical	Battery drainage attack	Active	Blacklisting nodes	Internal
Data link	Sybil attack	Active	Direct validation	Internal
Data link	Collision attack	Active	Use of hashing techniques	Internal
Data link	Replay attack	Active	Using timestamps on all messages	Internal
Data link	Traffic analysis	Passive	Encrypt traffic	Internal
Data link	Spoofing	Active	Packet filtering	Internal
Network	Selective forwarding attack	Active	Multi-hop acknowledgement	Internal
Network	Sybil attack	Active	Direct validation	Internal
Network	Hello flood attack	Active	Using signal strength for comparison	Internal
Network	Spoofing attack	Active	Packet filtering	Internal
Network	Wormhole attack	Active	Use of cryptography and GPS	External
Network	DoS attack	Active	Protecting endpoints	Both
Network	DDoS	Active	Network monitoring	Both
Network	Masquerading attack	Active	Code signing	Internal
Transport	Flooding attack	Active	Configuring firewall	Internal
Transport	Desynchronization attack	Active	Double authentication	Internal
Transport	DoS attack	Active	Protecting endpoints	Both
Transport	DDoS	Active	Network monitoring	Both
Transport	Man-in-the-middle attack	Active	Use of VPNs	Internal
Application	Spoofing	Active	Traffic filtering	Internal
Application	Resource	Active	Limit broadcasting	Internal

sexual diseases, infectious diseases and genetic information is derived using information linkage. This can result in privacy attacks on individuals and family health information [193]. The data linkage itself is a privacy threat, and it can also lead to other privacy problems like user profiling and data localization.

c) **Location Information:** This relates to the privacy of the physical location of the customers. Many personal wearable devices collect the users' current location information to send guidance or trigger specific contextual supports and services. The hackers who gain unauthorized access to the database could expose this information [194]. The location information can give clues regarding the places frequently visited by users and the typical occupancy timing of houses and office spaces. This can later be used to launch attacks or to conduct burglary.

d) **Information or Query Access:** This is related to the user's information from the database or the queries that the user initiates. The user's queries can give valuable information regarding the users' health status, medicines and treatments. Further, this information can also be combined with linked privacy attacks to extract information regarding relatives and their friends. This can reveal various habits and activities the user engages into and can be used for targeted advertising.

e) **Data Ownership:** Even though patient data holds a trove of vital information belonging to the patient, is the patient the sole owner of the data? Consider the case of vital signs of patient, imaging and investigation reports being collected at diagnostic centres; this data is retained with them for later use. Further, the doctors refer to these reports and prescribe medicines and treatments. It is evident that patient data is accessed and used by intermediaries, and thus, the patients sometimes don't even get to know who all have access to the data. Legislation must be made regarding data and patient data ownership regarding the secondary usage of data.

The importance of protecting privacy in medical IoT systems is more challenging and demanding, considering the data's sensitivity in the medical healthcare industry. There are risks associated with privacy when multiple features are integrated with a single medical IoT device. Data measurements can also be less accurate and error-prone, leading to users seeking unwanted treatments.

6.3   REVIEW OF EXISTING SOLUTIONS

Many significant works address the privacy and security issues of medical IoT. Most of the solutions have used conventional security solutions involving encryption, authentication and access control–based and blockchain-based solutions. We have reviewed the significant research works for security attacks in medical IoT devices in the following section.

6.3.1 MECHANISMS FOR SECURITY ATTACKS IN MEDICAL IOT DEVICES

Somasundaram et al. [181] reviewed and analysed various security issues for medical IoT devices and identified solutions to such problems. The security goal is to create a public infrastructure for device-level security, utilizing a mutually robust authentication scheme and a unique identity, a trusted public key infrastructure with a unique identity and a robust authentication scheme. This could be achieved by applying an advanced authentication mechanism, an authentication secured socket layer and lightweight cryptography. The goal is to achieve secure monitoring by increasing device security and identifying IoT devices' bizarre behaviour for continuous monitoring. This can be achieved by monitoring spatial information, temporal information, temperature monitoring and frequent device status updates in other devices in the network. The next level of IoT security is prevention; the motive is to prevent threats by protecting against external threats and preliminary detection of attacks; this can be achieved by monitoring incoming packets using a pocket-filtering firewall. Let's consider detection in the form of vulnerability management by identifying new vulnerabilities in IoT devices, improving IoT infrastructure security and detecting persistently. To conquer this goal, we can analyse data packets and monitor unusual data being transmitted. The next goal is to respond to the attacks by accessing system vulnerability, resolving implementation plan and preventing possible security dangers. To do this, we need to immediately update the faults of the device to other devices in the same network and after that avoid the readings from that compromised device.

In the following section, we investigated the different solutions for security attacks in medical IoT devices.

a) **Authentication Based:** Pankaj and Lokesh Chauhan [195] proposed to protect the network from various attacks using Secure Addressing and Mutual Authentication (SAMA) protocol. The proposed method uses a unique identification and addressing method for authenticating medical devices uniquely identified in a wireless IoT network. SAMA protocol also gives anonymity during the communication between the user and the medical server, with a session key. The authors claim that SAMA protocol protects against man-in-the-middle attacks, forward and backward secrecy, replay attack, malicious smart device deployment, privileged insider attack, device compromises, masquerade attacks, message forgery attacks and offline password guessing. Though the proposed system was tested using the AVISPA tool, Maria Almulhim and Noor Zaman [196] proposed a lightweight authentication system for medical IoT devices that was group based. This projected model used elliptical curve cryptography (ECC) principles to provide energy efficiency in medical IoT devices, mutual authentication and computations. The system creates a secure link between the sensor and the base station. The scheme would provide individual authentication to each node with a session key agreement. To save energy and cost, they use group authentication based on the distance between the base station and sensor nodes. The sensor node would collect the data and sent it to the head node, and the collected data would be forwarded to the server by the head node via the base station. The authors claim that their proposed system is secure against unknown key sharing attacks, impersonation attacks and man-in-the-middle attacks.

b) **Access Control Based:** Yang Yang et al. [197] suggested a self-adaptive access control method to preserve IoT healthcare devices' privacy. After encryption, the medical readings and files are transferred to the data store, which can be transferred to other users using cross-domain transfer protocols. While using traditional access control methods, only authorized personnel can access the patient's medical records. This creates excellent problems during a medical emergency. The patient needs to be provided with first aid, but the person providing first aid is unaware of the patient's medical history. This could lead to life-threatening complications. To overcome this, the authors offer a self-adaptive access control method, which incorporates giving access to authorized personal during regular times. Still, during a medical emergency, it gives a password-based break-glass mechanism. The proposed method also provides a de-duplication mechanism that removes all the duplicate files from the data store. The authors proved the system to be IND-CPA secure by solving the DBDH problem.

c) **Encryption Based:** Entao Luo et al. [198] gave a practical framework for collecting the patient's medical data and maintaining their privacy. They used Slepian–Wolf coding-based secret-sharing mechanisms that would secretly share the data and repair the damaged data. A distributed database is used for storing the data of the patient. So, when an authorized user asks for a patient's information, these multiple servers send the data without seeing through the content of the data. In the traditional methods of lossless operation using XOR for encryption, we need an initial vector (IV) and count pair. Attackers can easily guess the IV-counter pair and control the plain text leading to encryption and then decryption, giving access to the data. However, in this proposed system, a secrete key is given to the medical practitioner and the servers, so the attacker would not guess the IV without the key. Even if one of the many servers remains non-compromised, the patient's data will remain protected. The authors claim that they have tested their model against various attacks

Rafik Hamza et al. [199] gave a probabilistic cryptosystem that efficiently protects patient's privacy and protects key frame confidentiality. The system would also reduce energy consumption and the communication bandwidth. Traditional encryption algorithms for one-dimensional data and textual data cannot be used for medical data due to the digital data properties' limitations. Since the data is being transferred on exposed channels, there might be privacy loss of patients. The data being transferred must be encrypted to maintain the patient's privacy. The proposed system transfers images captured from wireless capsule endoscopy procedures using a prioritization method. The images generated after the encryption show behavioural randomness, which reduces the computational cost and brings high security. The proposed mechanism also processes the collected data without any leakage and allows only the authorized personnel to decrypt the data. The proposed method used a block symmetry encryption algorithm and tested using the NIST test, sensitivity, NPCR, UACI, histogram, information entropy, correlation coefficient, key space, image quality, time and performance. The proposed model is effective against statistical, differential and all-out attacks to find the secrete key.

The authors in [200] developed an encryption system using neural networks for transferring ECG data. A shallow neural network is used to remember the ECG pattern in few neurons. To consider the loss while converting to the neural network form, the authors encoded the loss into a small footprint with the help of Burrows–Wheeler transform (BWT), run-length encoding and move to front (MTF). For maintaining privacy in the network, only the neurons are encoded with the help of the session ID and session key, which is received from the health authority server every time the client wishes to transfer an ECG signal. The health authority server is only able to link the session ID to the patient. The health authority server would provide the doctor with the session key and session ID whenever the doctor wishes to see the reports and is authorized to do so. This proposed system reduces the size by 50%, giving a compression ratio of 6, reduces transfer time by 60% and ensures security.

Rihab Boussada et al. [190] proposed a novel solution for privacy preserving in medical IoT devices. The authors propose an identity-based encryption system (L-IBE) based on elliptical curve discrete logarithm (ECDL) problem, which defines public keys as user pseudonyms. This system provides authentication, data privacy, replay attack and data integrity. A build path algorithm (BPA) is used for communication, built on top of the L-IBE model. For validation and authentication, BAN logic and AVISPA tools are used. The proposed method is resistant to replay attacks, eavesdropping attacks, forging attacks, chosen messages indistinguishable and time correlation attacks. The proposed mechanism is tested for energy cost, storage overhead, computational cost and data transmission overhead.

d) **Blockchain Based:** Reyhane Attarian and Sattar Hashemi [201] proposed an anonymous protocol based on User Datagram Protocol (UDP) to protect privacy and data in a mHealth transaction. The proposed system uses onion encryption, onion network, onion routing and blockchain for transferring data. With the help of the identity disclosure process, the system can quickly identify malicious clients. Secure connections can be sent between two entities of the network without the need to transfer data. In this system, the client has a holding identity attribute (D) and other identity attributes (OD). After initial computations, the public and private keys are generated, and the data is sent to the verifier. The verifier verifies and authenticates D using the NIZKP of Goldwasser scheme and verifies the data OD. After verification, the data is signed and distributed on the blockchain. The admin or the health authority can register clients and ask them for their key using off-chain channels. Sending the data, they used an onion encrypted network that creates a chain between the client sending the data, onion nodes and the hospital. The hospital which receives the data verifies the identity of the sending client using the NIZKP of Goldwasser scheme. The signed and committed data is then received from the blockchain. If the receiver is authorized to receive the data, it will use the key it received from the off-chain anonymous onion connection. The commitment is then opened, and the data is stored in the local database. The proposed system is effective against calumniating attacks, pollution attacks, forgery attacks, repudiation attacks, omission attacks, eavesdropping attacks, replay attacks, impersonation attacks, collision attacks, man-in-the-middle attacks and Sybil attacks.

Alzubi et al. [202] used Lamport Merkle Digital Signature (LMDS) to make a highly secure system for IoT devices, assisted by blockchain. The model is authenticated using the Lamport Merkle Digital Signature Generation model by building a tree, where the leaf nodes signify the sensitive patient records' hash function. A centralized healthcare controller uses Lamport Merkle Digital Signature Verification to determine the root. In this process, the hash values of the public key and the root are compared; if the values are equal, it is the key's root, and the signature used is valid. This method identifies malicious users with minimum computation time and overhead. The proposed solution also reduces the struggle involved in the generation and storage of the signatures. It also uses large hash values, making it difficult for intruders and attackers to attack the system. The experimental results proved that the LMDS technique reduced the computational time and computations overhead by 25% and enhanced the security by 7%. Another advantage of the proposed system is that it does not require any trusted third party to exchange data; the blockchain efficiently performs the required computations.

6.3.2 MECHANISMS FOR PRIVACY ATTACKS IN MEDICAL IOT DEVICES

1. **User Data and Identity Information:** Data privacy is essential in every field, and it assumes greater significance when dealing with users' health information. The work done by Raaj Anand Mishra et al. [203] proposed a blockchain-based privacy-preserving and tamper-proof architecture for storing identity information for students. This brought a scalable storage mechanism, and authors have developed a proof of concept using the Ethereum blockchain. This work could also be extended to patient data, thereby controlling the patients' ownership and privacy. AttriChain, proposed by authors Wei Shao et al. [204] also uses blockchain-based technology to develop a distributed identity governance. This provides unlikability and anonymity to legitimate users and, at the same time, provides accountability to the actions of the users. The traceability of malicious activity is distributed in the network rather than relying on single identity management. The identity privacy is preserved in AttriChain using the user's signature created using user-generated transaction keys and self-generated transaction keys. No one, including the blockchain owners, can

derive the linkage between users and transactions committed by the users in this scheme. The sender's privacy is maintained by making a signature using attribute credentials rather than using public keys.

Another important work that focuses on privacy-preserving identity access management schemes is ARIES by Jorge Bernal Bernabe et al. [205]. The authors have used anonymous credential systems and identity protection leveraging the derived information from the users' personal information. The biometric data or any personal data collected from the user is not stored in clear text and is associated with anonymous identifiers. After the data is processed at the server, the biometric data is encapsulated in a biometric token signed and encrypted by the biometric service and sent to the user's device for storage. Thus, users' data is never stored at the server, enhancing the privacy of user data. As Wood in [206] described, building digital solutions with integrated identity management schemes is the need of the hour. There is a growing demand for identity as a service (IDaS) where user credentials and identity information can maintain users' privacy.

2. **Location-Based Privacy:** Many research works help in addressing the location-based privacy issues based on the protocol stack. One of the significant works done in this direction is [207], by using a technique to frequently dispose of the user's interface identifier at the media access control layer. The interface numbers of identifiers reveal the location information of the user. Another work that prevents location revealing is to associate two different IP addresses: static and dynamic. Also, security agents have been used to encrypt and route the messages in the network [208]. Another significant work done by authors in [209] is the query privacy algorithm based on spatial cloaking. In this technique, mobile users' location is mapped into a region of k-1 users to maintain anonymity. This approach helps keep the anonymity of the users' location and makes a user's query differentiable from another user's query. It has contributed significantly to anonymizing the continuous query.

The authors in [210] have developed an LP-Guardian solution for protecting the location privacy of android smartphone users using the concept of indistinguishability. This provides independent app protection and minimal user interaction. LP-Guardian provides location privacy in majorly three ways: the user's exact location is modified to the location coordinate of the centre of the city; routes traversed by users are modified to a synthetic route; and in cases where users require a higher degree of granularity, the location information is obfuscated. A cognitive approach utilizing existing network resources to ensure location privacy is introduced [211]. The multi-server architecture proposed by the authors blocks the direct connection between the location-based queries and the query issuers. The accurate query issuer's location is not included in the query that is sent to the server. The user's queries are sent to the server through the user's social media friends, and the query results are also sent to the user through trusted third-party applications. Obfuscation-based techniques protect users' location privacy in the research work done by C. A.

Ardagna et al. [212]. The data collected from user's applications or sensors is perturbed artificially to reduce the accuracy of location information. The obfuscation techniques used by the authors are of three categories: obfuscation by enlarging, shifting and reducing the radius. These techniques can be done individually or used in combination depending on the preference of the users. The advantage of this scheme is that obfuscation techniques can be chosen depending on the users' preference. A quantitative measure will also be given to the location privacy generated with the help of the algorithm.

3. **Data Linkage Privacy:** Linkage of data records can reveal vital clues regarding the health information of the individual and their relationships. Many health organizations use record linkage to derive meaningful insights from multiple data sources for epidemiological study and drug research. The authors in [213] have used the privacy-preserving record linkage technique, reducing the risk of disclosing information. They have used encrypted personal identifying information and probability-based linkage and have proven satisfactory results compared with traditional unencrypted personal identifiers. The privacy-preserving linkage techniques can separate identity information from medical records. The data holders can use passphrases to encrypt the personal identifiers. The authors' proposed work provides a significant milestone in privacy-preserving linkage information using the bloom filter method for approximate string comparisons. This technique has proven effective for data linkage without revealing private information and could greatly benefit drawing insights from data analysis. Few other significant research works preserve privacy and realize the full potential of the data. One among them is the secure, anonymous information linkage gateway [SAIL] done by Kerina H Jones et al. [214]. The gateway provides access to anonymous data and all analytical capabilities on the data. It is also responsible for different security features, including firewalls, encrypted network connections, two-factor authentication methods and security servers. It provides privacy-preserving the view and access of data-to-data users. Every data access request needs to be approved by the SAIL gateway after getting the signature of the data usage on the data access agreement. These techniques could be extended to be used in record linkage while maintaining data privacy. A comprehensive survey of privacy-preserving record linkage techniques is given in the research work by Dinusha Vatsalan et al. in [215]. Some of the techniques described by the authors include secure hash encoding, secure multi-party computation, pseudorandom functions, phonetic encoding, differential privacy, random values, etc.

4. **Data Access or Query Privacy:** Casper [216], the query processing for location services without compromising users' privacy, is a significant research in the direction of privacy-preserving query processing. The location anonymizer and privacy-aware query processor are the two integral components of this application. The user's location information is masked into spatial regions based on the privacy requirements. The privacy-aware query processor further processes cloaked spatial information instead of the exact location information.

In Casper, the original data is not stored; however, a perturbed version of the data is stored. Also, the location information of the user issuing the query is anonymized. This framework provides a privacy-aware query processor that provides a minimal and inclusive answer. Another critical research work in this direction is done by Yubin et al. [217] using data storage and query protocol based on homomorphic encryption. This preserves the privacy of both data owners and query users. The proposed solution is implemented using the Berkely database, a NoSQL database and the encryption and decryption process done by Elgamal and Paillier encryption system.

A new privacy-preserving query scheme called XRQuery [218] is proposed by Yekta et al. for fog computing–based IoT networks. The proposed technique can preserve privacy from the end-user's and service provider's perspective. The authors have evaluated the performance of the XRQuery mechanism and have demonstrated that the communication overhead is $O(logn)$, which is less than the existing protocol's efficiency of $O(n)$. This is also proven to be more computationally efficient than PQuery against which the algorithm is compared.

5. **Data Ownership Privacy:** The discussion of privacy issues of data ownership is very significant, and some of the essential works worth mentioning are described in this section. Nawaz et al. in [219] presented EdgeBoT, a framework using edge computing that provides data ownership. This performs P2P data trade without the need for a third party through a private Ethereum blockchain. The authors have used the ECC technique to encrypt the data, and a child key derivation function is used to generate a unique key every time. The authors have evaluated the performance and reliability of the model and found that the model uses only 40% of the computing power on average. Thus, this scheme is helpful for applications to be deployed on IoT devices and medical IoT devices. Another significant work that describes the importance of blockchain-based solutions for tracking the ownership of data is done by Jong-Hyung Lee et al. in [220]. They have pointed out that research in this direction can contribute to privacy and security challenges. However, they have rightly mentioned that research is in nascent stages that need to be fully evolved considering the inherent security challenges.

6.4 CHALLENGES IN EXISTING SOLUTIONS

The intrinsic nature of medical IoT devices in terms of computational power, memory and storage capacity is often overlooked when designing security and privacy solutions. Some of the critical research gaps in this direction are summarized below and in Figure 6.4.

a) All the solutions stated in previous sections were tested in a simulated system and not in real time. In real time, there can be multiple attacks happening at the same time. Once an attacker gets a way to enter the system, then it can send

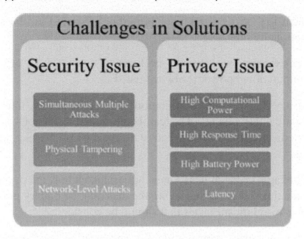

Figure 6.4   Challenges in solutions for security and privacy issues

various forms of attack, and the proposed systems are capable of handling all attacks at the same time with limited computational power, which is a matter of great concern.

b) Attackers can steal away specific sensors and may replace them with tampered sensors. It is possible that the tampered sensor sends false data or be spying on the patient with spying devices fitted in the sensor node.

c) Group authentication considered by many authors raises concerns. Since the network is divided into small groups, this can attract attackers to attack such networks.

d) Few authors provided authentication security, along with security from man-in-the-middle attacks and impersonation attacks. Still, these solutions do not consider network-level attacks like DoS, DDoS, and collision attacks. These attacks prevent the use of network resources, hence rendering the system useless.

e) Many works neglected malware attacks and DoS attacks. Homomorphic encryption schemes could be used to improve the efficiency of these cryptosystems further.

f) Few authors presented solutions to cyberattacks with blockchain help, but blockchains are not entirely secure; they are also vulnerable to time jacking, transaction malleability, routing and eclipse attacks.

g) While designing the solution for privacy issues, we should consider the intrinsic characteristics of medical IoT devices. Medical IoT devices have constraints in battery power, memory and processing power. Any potential solutions before being implemented should be evaluated in terms of the constraints of medical IoT devices and, very importantly, should not be a resource and computationally intensive.

h) Few privacy solutions solve the problem of query access privacy; however, their computational power is not evaluated.

i) Few privacy solutions have limitations in response time, thus restricting its use to static environments. This can be an impeding factor when used in dynamic medical environments when real-time data processing and analysis are required.

j) In data linkage, research works have not evaluated how the proposed solutions impact the time taken for retrieving the data and the battery power consumed. Latency is a significant factor that should be considered.

k) The techniques used to ensure identity and location-based privacy need to be evaluated for the usefulness of the information as most techniques use masking and obfuscation-based approaches.

Thus, solutions for security and privacy issues of medical IoT should be designed and implemented, focusing on the constraints of medical IoT devices and the usefulness and availability of patient data in the highly demanding dynamic environment.

6.5 CONCLUSIONS AND FUTURE SCOPE

We can witness an increased integration of technologies like AI, ML, image mining, AR and VR combined with the IoT in the medical domain. Many global healthcare service providers have started using IoT-Based solutions for their day-to-day operations and delivery. Combining the expectation of obtaining better and quality service from smart healthcare and achieving lower security and privacy compromise generates extensive interest. The concerns of security and privacy of medical IoT can deter the growth of this industry that can revolutionize the medical and healthcare sector. We have done a comprehensive survey of the progress of the medical IoT domain, prominent use cases, security and privacy challenges faced by smart healthcare applications. We have also reviewed important existing solutions for security and privacy attacks and the challenges in existing solutions. This review indicates that the way forward should be to increase the adoption of smart IoT devices in the medical field with privacy and security solutions in place suitable for resource-constrained medical IoT.

7 Security Concerns and Forensic Aspects of IoHT

Sitara K. and Manu.V.T.

CONTENTS

7.1 INTRODUCTION

In recent years, the healthcare industry has adopted connected technologies to more rapidly deploy next-generation medical devices and improve patient wellness. Most of such devices use software, including implantable units, diagnostic machines and monitoring equipment. The health technologies have amazing abilities to perform quick diagnosis, save lives and hence improve quality of life. Unfortunately, they also raise the alarming potential of inviting security misuse endangering patients.

Smart home appliances, hands-free digital assistants (SPA), environmental controls, security systems, door locks, etc., which bring control to our fingertips use

DOI: 10.1201/9781003239895-7

computing and connectivity to harness intelligence par human. The increased use of home monitoring video cameras and smart microphones in households, thanks to lower prices and the popularity of voice-activated gadgets, has introduced new vulnerabilities and security risks into the most private spaces in our lives. The worth of global digital health market was estimated to be 175 billion U.S. dollars in 2019. This figure is expected to increase 428% by 2025 to reach 660 billion dollars [221].

7.2 CYBER SECURITY

7.2.1 FOUNDATIONS OF SECURITY

The most accepted security model in cyber world is called CIA Triad, where C stands for confidentiality, I for integrity and A for availability. Confidentiality is maintaining information or data safe from unauthorized access. Integrity is maintaining the information or data without tampering; therefore it is authentic and reliable. Availability is maintaining the information or data for authorized access in a reliable and uninteruppted manner. Figure 7.1 shows the CIA Triad.

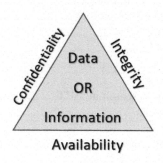

Figure 7.1   CIA Triad depicting the three principles as the edges of the data triangle

7.2.2 CYBER SECURITY TERMINOLOGY

- **Vulnerability** is a weakness in a system that can be exploited by someone to misuse the resources in it. It may be a known weakness or unknown till it is exploited. Most of the known vulnerabilities are indexed and explained on an online database called Common Vulnerabilities and Exposures (CVE).

- **Threat** is a potential circumstance which can cause harm to a resource.

- **Risk** is the impact of a threat on the asset or reputation of a system.

- **Attacker** is someone who maliciously exploits a vulnerability of a system and cause a threat to it by posing risks.

- **Attack surface** is a set of system elements where an attacker can brake into.

- **Attack vector** is those points on the attack surface that a potential attacker exploits.

- **Exploit** may be a set of instructions that help utilize the vulnerability in the system to gain access on an attack surface.

We have two contrasting sides of cyber security activities, which are attacker and defender. The former is a role which break into the system by exploiting the vulnerabilities and put it in risk. The latter attempts to protect or secure the perimeter of the attack surface. Both these roles demand constant understanding and evolution of the system according to the latest vulnerabilities and threats.

Defender side has an additional responsibility of suing the perpetrator in the court of law. Most of the cyber security breaches lead to risks and are considered a cyber-crime. The role and relevance of cyber forensics is on this defender side of cyber security domain as shown in Figure 7.2. A similar kind of diagram can be thought of on the attacker side.

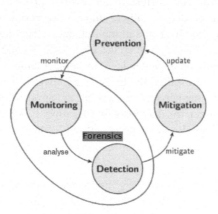

Figure 7.2   Defence side of cyber security of which forensics is a part, involves monitoring and detection of cyber security incidents.

A cyberattack is carried out by identifying the available vulnerabilities in a system. The steps are as depicted in the below diagram. The forensic procedure (Section 7.2.3) is followed at the evidence of the attacker's side from the delivery stage as shown in Figure 7.3. Here forensics can be applied on each of the modules of the attacker's activity. Collection and analysis of evidence from each module is integrated into a vector for preceding procedures.

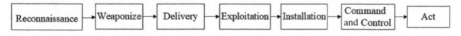

Figure 7.3   Attacker side of cyber security

7.2.3 CYBER FORENSICS TERMINOLOGY

An attack which occurs physically or virtually involves media which qualifies to be an evidence in the crime scene. This media happens to be at the attacker side as well as the defender side. The first and foremost aspect in forensics is how the evidence is treated.

Cyber forensics is the scientific collection and analysis of evidence so as to produce the findings as a report in the court of law. Cyber forensics is carried out in various steps like a) identification of evidence, b) preservation of evidence, c) acquisition of evidence, d) analysis of evidence and e) reporting.

As this chapter focuses on various devices ranging from sensors, network equipment to desktop computers, it is desired to have a fair understanding of each device's specific best forensic practices.

7.3 USE OF IoT ARCHITECTURE IN IoHT

An overview of the entire architecture of an IoHT is provided in accordance with the layered architecture of IoT. A subject under observation is fitted with sensors for the measurement of the physical and mental status. The data from these sensors is mostly heterogeneous. The layered architecture of IoT used in IoHT is shown in Figure 7.4. In the diagram, on the left side is the subject under observation. Wearable or implantable sensors are used on the body as a network. The data collected from these sensors is sent over the network and sent to the application and business layers for the medical practitioner for diagnosis and treatment. A similar architecture for Internet of Medical Things (IoMT) is proposed in [222].

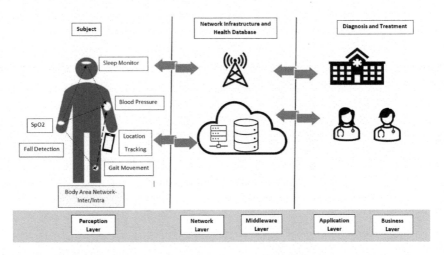

Figure 7.4   The layered architecture of IoT used in IoHT

The basic five-layer architecture of IoT is being used in IoHT, and the layers are described as below:

a) **Perception layer (PL)** is a set of interconnected or isolated sensors which are wearable or implantable in/on the subject's body and are used to directly or indirectly assess the health condition of the subject. In some cases, devices like cameras are used for visual inspection of the subject. The data like weight, room humidity, motion detection, room temperature, power consumption, location identification, detection of door closure, use and intensity of light, tracking location and posture, and person and object identification is measured with the deployment of this hardware. The hardware used in this layer can be classified into three [223] as follows, and the technologies used are also listed:

   a) **Personal Sensor Network** : RFID, LDR, pressure sensors, ultrasonic sensors, contact switches, hygrometer, etc.

   b) **Body Sensor Network** : Accelerometer, gyroscopes, GPS, ECG, EEG, EOG, EMG, PPG, etc.

   c) **Multimedia Devices** : CCTV, microphones, etc.

   The output data of each of these components varies, which poses challenges for integrating them for the subsequent layers.

b) **Network layer (NL)** is responsible for dealing with sending of data from various sensors through the network infrastructure for storing in the databases or cloud. Various network protocols are followed in this layer according to the requirement of the media and vendors. It also involves technologies like cellular networks, wireless LAN and various device-to-device communication strategies. Several network components are involved in the layer, like switches, routers and servers. On a security and forensic perspective, each of these components requires a very specific treatment. Both attackers and defenders have to check on the vulnerabilities in the protocols concerned. Zero-day attacks are a challenging concern for the defender side.

c) **Middleware layer (ML)** felicitates the integration of heterogeneous data collected from heterogeneous sensors. As discussed earlier, the output data formats may be numerical, time series data, categorical data or even analogue signal which is efficiently handled by the ML.

d) **Application layer (AL)** involves the presentation of the data processed in the previous layers, in a particular format which is interoperable across various health management softwares and algorithms. It manages applications like sending alert messages, mails, etc.

e) **Business layer (BL)** is related to how the consumers of the system get benefits out of the entire system. The layer deals with diagnosis, treatment, logistics of medicines, ambulance service, etc. Business decisions can be taken based on electronic health record (EHR). HL7 encoding produces a standard for the exchange of data with hospital information systems (HIS). It also helps maintain a life cycle of business processes by keeping track of the subjects, diagnosis information history, etc.

7.4   CYBER SECURITY IN IoHT

7.4.1   VULNERABILITIES

The Open Web Application Security Project (OWASP) [224] provides the list of top ten vulnerabilities for IoT, which are listed below. Description of the same is given below, explaining about the existence of each of these in the several layers of the IoHT architecture.

a) **Weak guessable or hardcoded passwords** are a vulnerability which is common for all the layers. Weak guessable passwords or hardcoded passwords occur in devices due to manufacturers' negligence. Such credentials are also found being shared on public platforms. The work in [225] discusses the use of reverse engineering to find such flaws like unauthorized device login by creating phantom devices.

b) **Insecure network services** affect the network layer only, but they may have side effects on the upper layers as well. The implementation of protocols can be vulnerable if they are not patched regularly. Even if security updates are released periodically, the system administrators concerned may not perform it due to several bottlenecks. The work [226] has summarized most of the present security threats related to this classification.

c) **Insecure ecosystem interfaces** are a interface-related vulnerability that occurs on all the layers. APIs are one such mechanism in this category whose vulnerability is of prime concern. Touch screen interfaces are vulnerable to reveal the fingerprints of users as discussed in [227]. Keystroke identification on smart devices for cracking into is shown in [228].

d) **Lack of secure update mechanism** Secure update mechanisms have to be automatic with security notifications to the system admin and users.

e) **Use of insecure or outdated components** is mostly on the lower layers as it occurs on hardware resources of IoHT. It arises as a part of cost-cutting strategy of the organizations.

f) **Insufficient privacy protection** is related to protection of privacy. Privacy was not a major concern during the initial days while developing IoHT. Therefore, the systems of the era deployed even now as mentioned as part of I5 may lead to data disclosures and put privacy at stake. The work [229] uses a secure communication using SIMON block cipher algorithm on sensed data on the PL, and to improve the privacy, a share generation model is used. The share generation uses an optimal user selection based on a metaheuristic algorithm called hybrid teaching and learning-based optimization (TLBO) algorithm. The generated copy of each ciphertext uses Chinese Remainder Theorem for sharing.

g) **Insecure data transfer and storage** is mostly taken care of using encryption techniques.

h) **Lack of device management** requires better management of the devices by a competent team, which is a must.

i) **Insecure default settings** Default settings are mostly well known across several public platforms.

j) **Lack of physical hardening** is a vulnerability that leads to taking control of the equipment physically. A systematic survey on various methods to protect hardware extraction of devices is provided by [230].

7.4.2 ATTACK SURFACES

Attack surfaces are spread across various layers of the IoHT architecture. They are identified in Table 7.1. The attack surfaces are identified as privacy, ecosystem, authentication, network traffic, device firmware, hardware (sensors), mobile application and device web interface [231].

An elaborate description of attacks and countermeasures on IoT are presented in [232].

Table 7.1
The Attack Surfaces on Various Layers

Attack Surface	IoHT Layer	Comments
Privacy	All	Important aspect for all layers as it is the primary concern
Ecosystem	All	Important aspect for all layers
Authentication	All	Important aspect for all layers
Network traffic	Network	
Device firmware	Perception	
Hardware (sensors)	Perception	
Mobile application	Application	
Device web interface	All	Important aspect for all layers

7.5 CUTTING-EDGE SECURITY RESEARCH IN IoHT

The work in [233] identifies the compromised device using an intrusion detection system before it gets several devices compromised in the network. The patterns of manipulations are identified using a deep sparse autoencoder network. The use of mobile agents is employed in [234] for intrusion detection for IoMT architecture which is scalable, fault tolerant and robust. Detection of device-level anomalies is done using polynomial regression. A healthcare testbed was created by the authors of [235], called the Enhanced Healthcare Monitoring System (EHMS). Along with network flow metrics, patient's biometrics were added as features in the creation of the testbed. Various machine learning algorithms were used to detect intrusion. The authors find it promising though the performance is not optimal.

The authors in [236] state that AI is feasible to secure IoT in four major risk factors like device authentication, DoS / DDoS attack defence, intrusion detection and malware detection. The work [237] elaborates healthcare sustainability via data security, privacy and AI's social acceptance. It ensures privacy of training data set through differential privacy and federated learning. It employs private blockchain-brokered entity for the aggregation of the global model gradients. Trustworthiness and provenance of the clients are ensured by blockchain technology. They introduce the terminology of explainability using deep learning process to ensure acceptability for a sustainable society. The authors created a data set in [238] called ECU-IoHT and a testbed. Common intrusion detection algorithms were tested on the setup with various well-known attacks.

7.6 IoT FORENSIC FRAMEWORKS

The history of forensic research is a relative new area in IoT or IoHT. To incorporate the diversity of evidence and challenges involved in forensic investigation, researchers have proposed many forensic frameworks and models [239]. But most of these were theoretical and moreover were not able to withstand the test of time with the evolving technological advancements. Considering the latter statement, it is to be noted that it is worthy to consider a few frameworks that have been proposed in the past five years. Also, we consider its relevance to the domain of IoHT.

1. **DFIF-IoT** is a generic forensic framework for IoT. Its full form is Digital Forensic Investigation Framework for Internet of Things. The framework adheres to the ISO standards in treating the evidence [240]. The authors introduce three modules – proactive, IoT forensics and reactive approaches. The proactive module is a precursor to incident identification. The IoT forensic model is in line with a work that introduces Forensics-aware IoT (FAIoT) [241]. Due to the adherence with the ISO standards, the evidence extracted using this framework has high probability of admissibility in the court of law.

2. **IoTDots** is a framework most suited for smart homes. It enables the collection of relevant evidence in accordance with the security policies laid out: anomalous activity recognition and malicious behaviour detection based on the data,

across the smart devices, apps and the ecosystem [242] IoTDoTs seems to be more of a practical approach than many other frameworks.

3. **PRoFIT** is a privacy-preserving framework in the investigation cycle in accordance with ISO/IEC 29100:2011 [243]. An extension of this work by incorporating the concept of digital witness is proposed in [244]. Digital witness [245] is any device that has the ability to collaborate in managing electronic evidence on technological and legal grounds. The framework looks for associated devices to understand the context of a crime scene. Privacy being a prime concern in IoHT, this framework can be considered a choice in the domain.

4. **Blockchain-Based Digital Forensic Investigation Framework**

   a) **FIF-IoT** uses blockchain technology to secure evidence, analysis and fact finding in crime incidents [246].

   b) **BIFF** utilizes blockchain technology for the entire treatment of evidence from collection to disposal phase [247]. Privacy of evidence submitter is preserved using a modified Merkle signature scheme.

   c) **Block-DEF** The work [248] proposes a digital evidence framework with the help of blockchain and presents a case study of file tampering. The scalable blockchain module uses a mixed blockchain design and an optimized name-based PBFT.

   d) **J. H. Ryu et al.** propose a blockchain-based decentralized investigation framework for IoT digital forensics [249].

   e) **Probe-IoT** proposes a design that ensures integrity, confidentiality, anonymity and non-repudiation of the evidence stored in the Bitcoin like public ledger [250]. Investigation of a crime incident using Probe-IoT facilitates acquiring of evidence from the ledger followed by verifying the authenticity and integrity of the obtained evidence.

7.7 FORENSICS IN IoHT

Forensic activities have to be carried out with an understanding of the attack surfaces and vulnerabilities on IoHT. A detailed study of various attack surfaces helps us to narrow down the search for attack vectors and therefore the exploitation of vulnerabilities.

The various steps of forensics are mentioned in Section 7.2.3. The initial stages focus mainly on the treatment of evidences. This is crucial as the mistake committed in identifying, preserving and acquisition of evidence will cause misjudgement of the crime incident. It leads to the analysis of wrong data which in turn leads to the wrong inferences.

IoHT has various layers as discussed in Section 7.3. The forensic approach on each of these layers is different as the type of data itself is different. All the forensic activities have to be separately performed on each of these layers. The challenges in dealing with the forensic aspects of IoT are discussed in [251].

7.7.1 FORENSICS IN PERCEPTION LAYER

The perception layer is considered the layer closer to a subject, as it is composed of various sensors for measuring health conditions, as discussed earlier. The data format of the measurement is either numeric, binary or time series data. As these data formats are trivial, the evidence can be dumped into a native one through available output interfaces and the analysis can be done with much each. But it is to be understood that the preservation and acquisition of the data can be difficult considering the volatility of the storage medium. Many of the devices used in this layer may not even have a storage medium itself, which makes the preservation and acquisition of evidence really hard and tricky. At times, however, after the identification of evidence, the later forensic steps become a challenging puzzle for the forensic investigator. Code injection attacks in this layer can be found in the literature, especially [252].

A firmware extraction technique is proposed in [230]. JTAG interface was used to identify the chipset and memory locations. This work was device specific and is effective when no traditional interfaces are available for logical acquisition. It evades evidence tampering through the use of the chip-off technique. A tool named OpenOCD is used in this approach [253]. The forensically relevant data stored on the devices in the layer can be acquired using a JTAG-based technique proposed by [254]. The authors propose an Internet of Things – Forensics Recovery Assistant (IoT-FRA) which tries to overcome the limitation of the former by incorporating more hardware models and prioritizing them in a forensic investigation.

7.7.2 FORENSICS IN NETWORK LAYER

Network layer involves various hardware and associated software components that help in sending the data obtained at the perception layer to the middleware for data integration. Abiding to network protocols is compulsory for each of these components so as to transmit or route data in a particular format. Each of the network components has to analysed using deep packet analysis or log analysis. Network packet capture of devices uses open-source tools like Wireshark [255] or tcpdump. A recent survey on various network forensic tools and techniques is discussed in [256]. Apart from packet capture analysis, log analysis of security devices deployed like intrusion detection system (IDS), intrusion prevention system (IPS), firewalls, etc., has to be analysed for abnormal activities.

Packet capture tools can be configured as man-in-the-middle (MITM), honeypot or similar setup. Taking the example of Wireshark [257], packets captured using the tool can be dissected to reveal its content in various layers of the Open Systems Interconnection model (OSI model). The content obtained is evidence of the crime incident. A testbed for IoT security is proposed in [258], and the authors have demonstrated the testing of smart thermostats and sockets using a GUI interface.

7.7.3 FORENSICS IN MIDDLEWARE LAYER

Middleware is the layer where the integration, storage and processing of data take place. This layer may be susceptible to script injection attacks for leakage or corruption of data. An example of middleware is Open Database Connectivity (ODBC), which is responsible for the communication between applications and database servers.

On a misconfigured ODBC connection arbitrary, queries can be executed against the database server through applications that use it to extract data. Trails of such unauthorized access leave trails of activity in log analysis, provided the perpetrator adopts an anti-forensic technique. Reverse engineering can be thought of as a solution for forensic evidence collection in this layer.

7.7.4 FORENSICS IN APPLICATION LAYER

Exploiting the vulnerabilities in the applications may be the cause of a crime in this layer. The perpetrator might have used application vulnerability scanners for reconnaissance before infiltration into the system. Active reconnaissance leaves forensic trails that can be detected and preserved as evidence for later stages of forensic activity. Passive reconnaissance may not leave forensic evidence in this layer, but in the network layer.

Infiltration may be done using penetration testing frameworks like Metasploit. The signatures of the exploits of such frameworks are well known from databases like VirusTotal [259], which makes it easy to understand the method of operation and collection of evidence accordingly. ExploitDB [260] is also a rich source of known vulnerabilities of softwares, along with its proof of concepts. It is interesting to note that such frameworks are used by naive hackers and white hackers.

Real hackers use custom-made payloads for exploiting the vulnerabilities of applications, making the job tough for forensic analysts. They may also use anti-forensic techniques like erasing trails of attack, thereby contaminating the potential evidence.

7.7.5 FORENSICS IN BUSINESS LAYER

Most of the forensic activities in this layer can be carried out using data analytics techniques. The business layer implements the decision-making of the entire IoHT setup; therefore, any activity that leads to hampering this may be recorded as evidence and analysed. The presence of malwares has to be inspected in this layer using anti-software solutions.

AI-based speakers are used to provide voice commands to the patients under observation in order to assist them in ambient living. Practices for data collection and investigation methods for various AI-enabled speakers are proposed in [261]. A similar work proposes forensics on an AI speaker that supports display, namely Echo Show [262].

7.8 RECENT WORKS

In a healthcare facility, the subjects are provided assistive technologies like smart plugs, voice assistance devices, etc., to ease their physical constraints. We have identified a few forensic and security-related research articles in recent times in the literature.

Smart Plug is a plug which can be automated remotely by a smartphone app for scheduling appliances. Buffer overflow attacks on such devices are reported in [263] and [264] by the researchers at MacAfee. The authors in [265] have experimentally analysed forensic artefacts from five major such devices using various network setups. They encountered various challenges like rooting of devices, heterogeneous file formats, encryption algorithms, need for reverse engineering and logging in the cloud than device itself.

The doctoral thesis by [266] has done various security and penetration testing on smart devices like Amazon-Echo-Dot v3 and Google-Home-Mini, followed by a forensic analysis. The limitation as expressed by the author was that the devices under consideration have limited web browser interface. Due to this limitation, it was not able to acquire physical dumps of the devices under forensic analysis.

Voice commands given to Alexa's API were studied by [267]. They discuss how data is stored at multiple places and throw light on counter anti-forensic techniques on such devices. Anti-forensic activities deliberately done on smart devices are performed and later exposed in [268].

The work in [269] tries to reduce the complexity of forensic approaches in IoT ecosystem by introducing the terminologies of DNA and genes to uniquely identify the devices under investigation. It involves the concept of an IoT forensic server, which is still under implementation at the time of writing this article. A framework for smart home forensics is proposed in [270], in which the authors work with data from Google Nest Hub, Samsung SmartThings and Kasa Cam. The forensic activities are listed in Table 7.2 along with the difficulties in performing them. Tick marks indicate that the activity is easy.

Table 7.2
Forensic Activities

Forensic Activity	PL	NL	ML	AL	BL	Comments
Evidence identification	✓	✓	✓	✓	✓	Evidence can be identified from all these layers. It is challenging in PL as there may not be a storage device. Data may be directly uploaded to upper layers.
Evidence preservation	Hard	✓	✓	✓	✓	Depends on the volatility of the media in each of these layers
Evidence acquisition	Hard	✓	✓	✓	✓	The concept of cloning on similar media is impractical.
Evidence analysis	✓	✓	✓	✓	✓	From higher layer to lower layer, the amount of data increases.
Inference generation	✓	✓	✓	✓	✓	Difficulty is fairly the same across various layers.
Presentation	✓	✓	✓	✓	✓	Difficulty is fairly the same across various layers.

7.9 CONCLUSIONS

Cyber security is a prime concern for health sector as the data is sensitive. We discussed the constituents of IoT in detail along with IoHT. Details about each of the layers in these were given. A taxonomy of cyber security and cyber forensics was elaborated. Considering both these aspects of security and forensics, we have identified the attack surfaces based on the layered architecture along with the OWASP top ten vulnerabilities on each. We discussed how the OWASP top ten vulnerabilities can be found in IoHT, citing the literature on IoT. A section is devoted for the discussion of cutting-edge research in the domain of IoHT security. We reviewed various IoT forensic frameworks in the recent literature. Forensic aspects in each of the IoHT layer were discussed. Recent works in smart devices in the domain of security and forensics are presented thereafter.

We understand that there is no practical framework that can scale over the variety of device architectures and heterogeneous data formats, though each of the discussed frameworks performs well within their constraints. There exist lots of open challenges, mainly in forensics, especially the treatment of evidence from identification to analysis. The equipment vendors follow a closed source or proprietary approach to protocols, APIs and algorithms. Research in this domain will be more productive if there are open source frameworks and standards with privacy preservation and security. Threat-reporting platforms have to be established for medical equipments, and the users have to actively participate in keeping pace with attack mitigation steps.

Regulatory bodies have to be established to enforce the periodical updation of hardware and software that are found vulnerable through periodic security audits. Forensic readiness has to be enforced by such bodies so that if in case there is an incident, the investigation team will get its initial thrust in the proceedings.

Encryption plays an important role in preserving privacy and confidentiality of data. But it is observed that cryptographic schemes are neglected due to power consumption involved in computation. The latest sensor hardware is found to be consuming less power, and there are evolving lightweight cryptographic algorithms that can be incorporated in IoHT. Compromising powerful cryptographic schemes for powerful processing units is not desirable these days.

In designing smart homes or spaces with ambient, assistive living using artificial intelligence, neglecting security will not only defeat the purpose but also cause harm. Therefore, at each level of architecture, proper care should be taken to safeguard the data and information.

☆ ☆ ☆ ☆

8 Recent Security Issues and Countermeasures on IoHT

Misbah Shafi and Rakesh Kumar Jha

CONTENTS

8.1 INTRODUCTION

In recent years, *Internet of Healthcare Things (IoHT)* has enticed a lot of recognition in the applications of the medical domain. The healthcare systems make use of wireless communication network (WCN) to coordinate medical devices and individuals, thereby facilitating the medical particulars. The primary support of the IoHT is to monitor the status of the patients remotely and diagnose them more accurately. In terms of cost, it is expected to save approximately 300 billion USD annually [271–273].

In view of the current outbreak of the global pandemic COVID-19, the use of IoHT can prove an efficient way to monitor patients remotely especially for the individuals requiring emergency assistance. The IoHT reduces the requirement of face-to-face consultation by using smart diagnostic devices and therefore improves the quality of life care. The advent of artificial intelligence (AI) in IoHT with semantic knowledge and sensing ability offers dynamic scheduling, telemedication, home care and monitoring. The systems of IoHT employ medical devices and services to improve the experience of the end-user like optimum time management, source management, service management and diagnosis management [274]. The development of IoHT is considered as one of the powerful paradigms that have raised the standard of living all around the globe. However, the parameter of security is one of the major challenges in the field of IoHT and occupies the utmost importance. Inadequate security offers consequences such as compromised privacy, attacks causing delayed

DOI: 10.1201/9781003239895-8

disruption, eavesdropping and unauthorized access. The IoHT requires protection at different stages such as data monitoring, data collection, data transmission, diagnosis and storage [184, 275, 276].

8.2 SECURITY SOLUTIONS IN THE LITERATURE

Various traditional security solutions were followed to satisfy the security requirements of IoHT. However, due to the system requirements such as power consumption, ultra-low latency, reliability and accuracy, traditional security solutions do not guarantee appropriate and absolute security. Alladi et al. in [277] suggest a two-stage authentication protocol to enhance the physical security in IoHT network against node replacement and node tampering attacks. Three types of nodes are considered in this network viz. a patient node, a sink node and the server node. The patient node initiates the process of authentication from the healthcare cloud server via the sink node. The scheme follows two stages of authentication. The first stage occurs between the sink and the server node. The sink node and patient node perform the second stage of authentication.

The authors in [278] analysed the security performance of the IoHT network using convolutional neural network (CNN) prediction model. The model consists of four convolution layers and the four inception branch blocks. The model extracts data features of the available healthcare data. The model analyses the security performance using secrecy outage probability (SOP). The mean squared error of the scheme is reduced by 20%.

In view of security in the data collection of IoHT systems, a mechanism of secret sharing and data repairing is provided in [198]. The sharing scheme involves Slepian–Wolf coding where multiple cloud servers are employed for the storage of data. These servers offer collaborative construction of patient data sharing with the healthcare profession with a patient access control methodology. The authors in [279] observed secure data collection by using the KATAN secret cipher algorithm in IoHT. The network is divided into four layers. The first layer is the Internet of Things (IoT) network sensors. The second layer is the fog layer. The third layer is the cloud computing layer and the healthcare provider in the fourth layer. The hardware-based cipher algorithm and the secret cipher share algorithm are the two techniques included in the first two layers. The KATAN algorithm is based on secret cipher sharing and is used to provide data privacy. To provide security to the patient's personal data, a distributed database technique is used at the cloud computing layer. The authors in [280] enhanced the security and privacy of the healthcare data collection using the signature technique. The noise is added to the healthcare data to improve privacy.

Ding et al. in [281] employed an edge server for data authentication and data integrity verification. Privacy is ensured by the encryption of health data before transmission to the edge server. The cloud server performs decryption to certify data availability. The authors in [272] enhanced the security in IoHT through the methodology of identity management. The technique involves the mapping of the credential information of the user. The attribute-based encryption using the hash technique is used to parse the information of the user's credentials. The output token during account creation is formulated using elliptic curve cryptography (ECC). Further, the key verification identity management is executed in the fog node. The authors in [282] analysed the password-based security vulnerabilities using a password strength evaluation mechanism. The method includes the personal information of the user to estimate password strength and hence chooses the password having a higher level of security.

Wang et al. in [283] evaluated the security framework, Identified Security Attributes (ISA), for the IoHT network. The scheme uses an analytical hierarchical process and Technique for Order Preference by Similarity to Ideal Solution (TOPSIS). The framework consists of two processes. The first process involves the derivation of weight attributes using an analytical hierarchical process, and the second process involves the evaluation of security criteria using TOPSIS methodology. Islam et al. in [284] improved the security in IoHT by using the mechanism of blockchain. The health data is attained by the users through the unmanned ariel vehicle (UAV) such that the data is stored at the nearest server. The authentication follows two processes. The first process is encryption, and the second is the blockchain. The UAV establishes the communication with body sensor hives by using tokens and then communicates the shared key. The UAV then stores the health data by using blockchain.

Similarly, the authors in [285] securely transmitted the healthcare images using a cryptosystem based on the trigonometric map design. The cryptosystem generates the first three keystreams set from the latest trigonometric map to calculate hamming distance. The concept of bit XOR is applied on the output distance vector with the keystream. The Mandelbrot set is defined as the shift algorithm for the pixel shuffling. The resultant vector and the output from the earlier process are bit XORed to obtain the encrypted image. The authors in [286] performed trust evaluation based on the mechanism of artificial neural networks. The degree of trust is evaluated by aggregating the evaluation of parameters such as compatibility computation, packet delivery calculation, and node identity, which are trust computations of reliability. The mechanism follows the combined mechanism of ECC and secure hash algorithm for the encryption scheme. The other recent methodologies for the enhancement of security in IoHT are given in Table 8.1.

8.3 OPEN CHALLENGES IN THE SECURITY OF IOHT

There are various challenges identified in the security of the IoHT network that are required to be addressed [181, 276, 301–307], and are discussed below:

a) **Latency:** The huge healthcare data volume creates a drastic impact on the latency. Moreover, the IoHT involves end-to-end processing and transmission, which increases the delay in the network. Several security enhancement mechanisms were defined in IoHT. Besides, creating a balance between latency and security is still an open challenge. Therefore, security schemes especially for time-critical applications such as telesurgery are required to fulfil the demand of security with minimum latency.

Table 8.1

Recent Security Enhancement Methodologies in IoHT

Ref	Technique/Scheme	Objective	Target Parameters	Target Attacks	Network Type
[287]	Improved CLAS	To enhance security using CLAS for WMSN	Computational time and communication cost	First message attack	Healthcare WMSN
[288]	Smart service authentication	To enhance mutual authentication protocol for TMIS using cloud environment	Computational time	Health report revelation attack, server spoofing, denial of service (DoS), stolen smart card attack, and non-repudiation	Medical healthcare system network
[289]	Boneh-Franklin identity-based distributed decryption scheme	To design a lightweight decryption scheme while maintaining the security	Time consumption	Ciphertext attack	Electronic personal healthcare system
[290]	Blind batch encryption scheme	To obtain an optimized balance between privacy and security	Time cost	Collision attack, external attack, reuse attack, man-in-the-middle (MIM) attack, replay attack and privacy attack	Smart healthcare system network
[291]	Fuzzy commitment scheme	To resist against mobile device loss attack	Time cost	Stolen smart card attack, mobile device lost attack and impersonation attack	Wireless medical sensor network systems
[292]	Blockchain-based trust management technique	To enhance the secure communication between the patients and healthcare professionals	Trust value	Insider attacks	Medical smartphone networks
[293]	SDN	Security improvement in data sharing healthcare systems	Response time	Identity theft attack and insider attack	Data sharing healthcare system networks
[234]	Mobile agent–based ID scheme	High accuracy-based intrusion detection	Detection accuracy and energy usage	DoS, data falsification and fabrication, and privacy attack	Internet of Medical Things (IoMT)
[294]	Mosaic gradient perturbation scheme	To enhance the privacy and deteriorate the risk of model inversion attack	Accuracy and time computation	Model inversion attack	Smart healthcare system network
[295]	Anomaly intrusion detection	Detecting illegal behaviour using machine learning (ML)	Accuracy and time cost	Replay attack, malware attack and shoulder surfing attack	Medical IoT system networks
[296]	Additive homomorphic encryption scheme	To improve secure monitoring in wireless IoT-Based body sensors	Computation time	Chosen plaintext attack and weekly unforgeable attack	Wireless body sensor networks
[297]	Blockchain scheme	To ensure secure data transmission	Verification error and cost of witnessing	MIM attack	Body area networks
[298]	Elgamal blind signature technique	To develop a privacy-preserving scheme for searching medical records	Execution time	Violent ergodic attacks	IoMT
[299]	Hash functions and XOR operations	To develop a secure data communication mechanism between the devices in healthcare IoT	Latency, communication time and energy of sensor devices	Replay attack, forgery attack, de-synchronization attack, attacks on availability, key agreement, mutual authentication and untraceability	IoMT
[300]	One-way hash function and bitwise XOR operation	To develop an anonymity-preserving authentication mechanism	Computational cost	Replay attack, DoS attack and MIM attack	Digital health networks

b) **Complexity in security schemes:** Complexity is one of the challenging parameters in IoHT. Moreover, the employment of the security methodologies such as cryptographic techniques in IoHT increases the complexity of the network. The complexity affects the storage capacity, resource consumption, availability, quality of service and process management of the IoHT network. Therefore, an efficient security mechanism for the IoHT with low complexity is required to be developed.

c) **Real-time security status:** The security of the IoHT network is required to be examined continuously such that the status of the security remains up-to-date. However, continuous examination of the whole network is a cumbersome process and requires more battery consumption. Besides, determining the security status of the network at regular intervals can pose a security threat in the IoHT network. Therefore, real-time security examination of the IoHT network is an open issue and requires to be optimized.

d) **Accuracy and computation time:** It is considered as one of the primary parameters of the security mechanisms based on AI. It defines the correctness of the security mechanism, such as in intrusion detection schemes, the appropriateness of distinction between the valid node and an invalid node is defined by the accuracy. Maintaining a high accuracy with a big volume of data for the existing attacks is a considerable threat required to be addressed.

e) **Limited resource:** The IoHT involving body area network relies on a limited power such that the energy incorporated during processing is less. The wearable IoHT devices are required to have sufficient power to execute for a longer duration. Especially for IoHT-based implants, the required active time is preferably longer as the replacement of them is painful and costlier. Moreover, the size of the IoHT is comparatively small with restricted memory and limited power. Security mechanisms are required to execute with small power and memory. The current security schemes are large, and to operate well with constraints is quite challenging.

f) **Heterogeneity:** The IoHT involves a wide variety of applications. These applications encompass a wide variety of device classes. The devices vary in properties and exhibit different regulatory requirements. Applying the same security mechanism on different classes of devices is likely to create an adverse impact on the security of the network. Therefore, specific application-based security schemes are required to be suggested.

g) **Mobility management:** The devices in IoHT are operated in a dynamic environment. Mobility plays an important role in the security of the communication network. The interferences due to mobility create distracted communication which ultimately affects the security of the network. Furthermore, the IoHT occupies a diverse nature of mobility speeds. Considering different mobility speeds while analysing security is an important challenge and is required to be addressed. Therefore, security schemes with the consideration of the varying mobility in the IoHT network are desirable.

h) **Resiliency:** The security schemes are required to be resilient such that the errors in the mechanism are not able to create a drastic impact on the decision. The schemes are required to be able to recover the error at a high pace without any effect on the network of IoHT. Designing the security schemes with the property of resiliency is an open challenge.

i) **AI-based attacks:** AI-based attacks in the IoHT network are a new research direction that requires immense attention. The application-specific attacks based on AI in IoHT can create a serious threat wherein minute disturbances devised by the attacker on the devices of the network can prove extremely catastrophic. Therefore, countermeasure strategies for such attacks are required to be formulated.

j) **Intrusion prevention schemes:** The security of the IoHT can be improved by the methodology of intrusion prevention schemes. These schemes are required to be able to eliminate the effect of the attacker and continue the function of the system without failure. Moreover, a security mechanism must be capable of enhancing the security of the network and counterattacking the detected intruder. However, based on the tiny protocol stack, the adaptation of the intrusion prevention or security enhancement schemes is an open challenge.

8.4 CASE STUDY: REAL-TIME SECURITY PERSPECTIVE OF IOHT (FITNESS TRACKER) BASED ON MOBILITY

The devices execute differently in the state of mobility, thereby creating a vulnerable threat in the security of the IoHT network, for example in the case of the fitness tracker. The security scheme proposed for the fitness tracker in the state of rest creates a variation in the performance of the tracker in mobility [308]. The case study based on the performance analysis of the fitness tracker is analysed in this section. The fitness tracker in the body area domain of IoHT continuously monitors the movement of the body. The movement is observed by the three-axis accelerometer. Collection of data takes place all the time as the device is powered up on a human body. The device keeps track of an individual while the individual is in the state of standing, walking or running. The data is further analysed either on the device itself or on the monitor with which the tracker is connected and synced.

The tracker device works on the principle of step count. The step count is then multiplied by the stride to estimate the walked distance. For the improved accuracy of the emergency-based healthcare applications or the specific healthcare patients such as patients with heart diseases, the devices make use of the GPS to calibrate it with the stride of the individual. The calibration with the GPS requires several minutes of walking at a constant pace. Further, certain fitness trackers provide the liability to enter the starting and end points and even the stride to calculate the performance.

However, the smart tracker devices automatically detect the different postures and consequently show the performance. The analysed data is then stored for the required further processing or future reference or is communicated to the synced device.

This case study is based on the data collection of the device while analysing the state of mobility. Most of the security mechanisms devised for the IoHT network do not incorporate the concept of mobility. The healthcare data can be affected drastically even by the small movement of the body area wearables of the IoHT network. Taking advantage of the fluctuations in the data, the attacks based on data authentication and data integrity can be compromised. A few of the current IoHT-based projects are summarized in Table 8.2.

Table 8.2

Current Internet of Healthcare Things Projects

S.no.	Project Name	Aim of the Project
1.	Transforming healthcare with 5G [309]	Advancement of remote diagnosis and the development of robotic-assisted surgery
2.	Healthcare IoT solutions [310]	To develop energy-efficient healthcare IoT-Based systems
3.	AI-powered synchronized stroke care (Viz pager) [311]	AI-based healthcare monitoring system
4.	Re-imagining the possible in the Indian healthcare ecosystem with emerging technologies [312]	To upgrade the healthcare industry in coordination with the emerging networking systems
5.	Smart e-health gateway [313]	To develop IoT-Based healthcare systems
6.	Deliver intelligent, connected healthcare [314]	To provide real-time-based healthcare using cloud technology
7.	Smart Autonomous Robotic Assistant Surgeon [315]	To develop a surgical robotic system based on next generation communication to implement robotic minimally invasive surgery
8.	Medtronic's robotic-assisted surgery [316]	To develop a digital robot-assisted surgery system
9.	DOBOT Magician [317]	To develop a lightweight, intelligent robotic arm

8.5 RECENT SECURITY ISSUES IN IOHT

With the recent advancement in the IoHT, a plethora of security issues and a lack of efficient security mechanisms have created a threat in the domain of healthcare. The dependency on the smartphones, sensor readings, biometric data of patients, wearable devices, cloud storage and complex algorithms has introduced vulnerable menaces in the security of IoHT [318–322]. The recent security issues in the IoHT are addressed in this section as follows:

a) **Password management flaw:** Password is considered as the primary security aspect to protect against the misuse of the concerned records of the patients. Using weak password is one of the main concern that can affect the security of the data. The use of weak password by the patient or the concerned health authority can be detected by the brute force. Further, the use of the computers with stored password also creates a vulnerability to various attacks such as hijacking, masquerading, jamming and DoS. Another possible threat with password mismanagement involves the reuse of passwords with multiple websites and programs. The use of similar passwords by the patient on multiple websites can lead to a threat to the security of the IoHT. To address this issue with the IoHT devices, patients and the concerned authorities should secure the network with unique passwords.

b) **Weak update management:** The integrated use of different devices in the IoHT creates connectivity with ease of use. However, with time, the devices become more exposed to the attackers and create a security threat to the whole network as well as to the life of the patient. Weak update management may lead to the issues such as delay, less accuracy and less efficiency, which ultimately affects the security of the network. Therefore, the devices are required to be updated by the latest security models to detect the newest bugs and prevent the attacks.

c) **Interfaces with incompetent security performance:** The interface forms the primary parameter to the applications and external service, although a well-integrated interface assists the services and benefits the overall system. However, the use of cloud and web services exposes confidential information such as keys to the third-party applications. Therefore, it creates threats in terms of attacks on confidentiality such as DoS, pharming attacks and phishing attacks.

d) **Inadequate data security:** One of the significant concern in the security of IoHT is the security of the data and records of the patients. The continuous data obtained from the patients creates an impact on the decision of the recovery of the patients. The compromised devices in the IoHT provide access to the confidential information of the patients, thereby creating a threat to data security.

e) **Improper security management:** The improper management of connected devices in the domain of IoHT reveals drastic number of attacking risks and

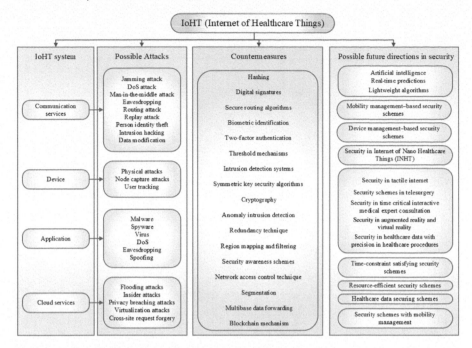

Figure 8.1 Security-based visualization of the IoHT

vulnerabilities. Improper security management includes unauthorized access to the devices connected in the network, utilizing unconfirmed legacy operating systems, echo device-supported surveillance equipment integrated with the main healthcare network, unawareness of the active smart objects in the network, improper device security monitoring and continuous support of the devices to the security requirements. The possibility of the ransomware attack, disrupted operations, loss of information and reputational damage is increased by the issue of improper security management. Additionally, the visualization of security in IoHT is shown in Figure 8.1

8.6 CONCLUSIONS AND FUTURE RESEARCH DIRECTIONS

Security in wearable healthcare systems is an emerging field and requires more advancement. Security in data acquisition and storage based on cloud technologies is another research direction in IoHT. Data processing, algorithm efficiency and AI for the enhancement of the security of IoHT can prove extremely valuable.

☆ ☆ ☆ ☆

9 Future Wireless Communication Systems to Enable IoMT Services and Applications

Francisco Falcone, José Javier Astrain,
Idoia Aguirre, Jesús Daniel Trigo and Luis Serrano

CONTENTS

9.1 WIRELESS COMMUNICATION SYSTEMS

The Internet of Medical Things (IoMT) market has grown exponentially from double-digit values, approximately USD 41.2 billion, during the past decade to three figures, USD 158.1 billion, in the present decade [323]. This growth can have its pillars in two aspects. On the one hand, it is a new idea of patient empowerment given that daily clinical practice can spin around them with IoMT. This concept can include not only common medical devices equipped with connectivity but also wearable devices, as well as apps connected to the hospital information system, even including more complex devices such as drones or artificial intelligence (AI) and augmented reality algorithms [324–326]. On the other hand, the availability of technology and the past, present and future scenario of COVID-19 have led to the deployment of health services based on IoMT where the efficiency of the system and the safety of both the patients and the health workers and, therefore, security in the provision of these 'new'

DOI: 10.1201/9781003239895-9

health services prevail. This evolution requires to consider additional implementation aspects, such as seamless/continuous connectivity, data/system interoperability, availability of distributed data/cloud handling infrastructure as well as user/data security and privacy.

One of the key aspects in order to enable the required interactivity levels that define context aware scenarios and their related applications is communication systems, as a part of the information and communication technology framework. In this sense, communication networks have experienced a sustained evolution towards network convergence, with the goal of providing the most adequate resource allocation given quality of service/quality of experience metrics [327–329]. Wireless communication systems are largely employed within general Internet of Things (IoT) and more specific IoMT applications, owing to their ease of deployment, ubiquity, mobility and scalability. There are multiple wireless communication systems that can be employed, given coverage/capacity requirements (i.e. maximum transmission rate for given receiver sensitivity values), as well as by constraints such as limited energy availability, ergonomics, form factor or low cost, among others. Moreover, in the case of IoMT applications, there can be inherent requirements in relation to node/sensor location within the user, requiring intra-body or inter-body communication capabilities. Wireless communication systems can be classified depending on there coverage range, as well as their mobility level, into the following categories:

a) **Wide area networks (WAN)** provide worldwide coverage levels, with high mobility. Public land mobile networks (PLMNs) and satellite communication networks (SatCom) are the main WAN types. Current PLMNs provide heterogeneous operations (given by variable cell size as well as by network exchange via hand over mechanisms), co-existing legacy 3G networks, mature 4G networks and 5G networks in rollout phase. The evolution of 5G networks gives rise to the concept of beyond 5G (B5G) and future 6G networks, which are expected to be a reality by 2030. PLMNs usually operate below 6 GHz frequency range (mainly in 900 to 3600 MHz range), whereas SatCom usually operate in X-band. 5G networks have opened the path to the use of millimetre wave spectrum, mainly in the 26–28GHz bands, whereas future 6G systems are exploring more intensive use of sub THz frequencies, particularly up to 300 GHz frequency range [330].

b) **Low-power wide area networks (LPWANs)** provide coverage levels of up to several km with respect to the corresponding gateway. LPWANs have gained popularity, as a natural evolution of wireless sensor networks, focusing on providing extended battery life (up to 10 years, taking advantage of energy-harvesting techniques, such as photoelectric cells, thermoelectric effects, piezoelectric effects or electromagnetic energy scavenging via rectenna elements, among others). Within LPWANs, different systems have been developed mainly within the framework of the 802.15 standard, such as LoRa/LoRaWAN, SigFox, ZigBee or eNocean, among others. PLMN-based networks oriented towards telemetry/sensor networks can also be considered a part of LPWANs, including systems such as NB-IoT or LTE Cat M.

Transmission rates are in general below 250 kbps, operating in frequency bands in the 400 Mhz to 2400 MHz frequency range.

c) **Wireless local area networks (WLANs)** were developed in the late 90s as the wireless evolution of Ethernet 802.3 standard and has become one of the most employed access networks, providing coverage levels usually below the km range. WLANs are developed within the IEEE 802.11 standards framework, providing transmission rates that vary from 1 Mbps to over 10 Gbps in the case of 802.11ax (referred as Wi-Fi 6 standard). WLAN frequency bands have been allocated from sub 1 GHz bands (in the case of 802.11ah, focused on IoT applications, in the 900MHz band) up to millimetre waves (60 GHz band in the case of 802.11ad). The most employed currently are in the 2.4 GHz and 5.5GHz to 5.9 GHz frequency ranges (being the upper band of the latter reserved mainly for vehicular communications).

d) **Personal area networks (PANs)** were also developed within the framework of 802.15 (mainly 802.15.4) and provide short-range communications (below 100m) usually for a limited time, enabling connectivity of multiple types of devices, such as wearables to mobile gateways, such as smartphones. Examples of PANs are Bluetooth and Bluetooth Low Energy, operating in the 2.4 GHz frequency, with transmission rates usually in the 1–2 Mbps range as well as ultrawideband (UWB) technology, which operate in the 4 GHz and 6 GHz frequency bands.

A schematic view of the coverage/capacity relations provided by wireless communication systems, spanning between PAN, LPWAN, WLAN and WAN, is depicted in Figure 9.1, and their characteristics are described in Table 9.1.

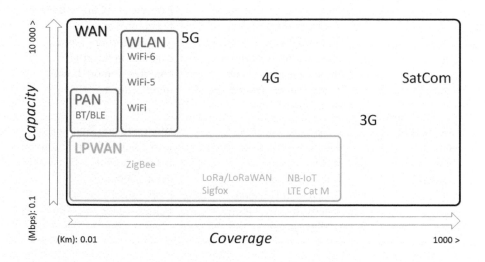

Figure 9.1 Schematic overview of coverage/capacity relations for different wireless systems, from LPWAN to WAN

Table 9.1
Wireless Networks' Overview

System	System Parameters	Application
Public land mobile networks	Wide area network, high mobility, wide area coverage and operation frequencies from UHF to mm-Wave. Tx speeds from kbps to 10 Gbps (5G NR FR2)	2G to 5G systems, employed for high mobility combined with high data rate requirements. Remote patient monitoring and remote assistance/ diagnostics
Wireless local area networks	Local area network, room to campus area connectivity, operation frequencies in the 2.4 GHz, 5.5 GHz, 60 GHz and in sub 1 GHz IoT bands (IEEE 802.11ah). Tx speeds from 1 Mbps to 10 Gbps (802.11ax)	Wi-Fi systems. Can be used for local connectivity of medical instrumentation, remote assistance/ diagnostics and electronic health record handling
Low-power wide area networks	Wide area network, low mobility, extended area coverage (in the range of 10 km–20 km, depending on scenario). Operation frequencies in the sub 1 GHz range; low Tx speeds in the kbps range	LoRa/LoRaWAN, SigFox, ZigBee, etc. Can be used for telecontrol and telemonitoring of assets, for example in hospital complex, remote home monitoring, etc.
Body area networks, personal area networks	Constrained coverage, usually within the range of metres. Operation frequencies mainly in the 2.4 GHz ISM bands. Tx speeds in the 1 Mbbps to 3 Mbps range	Bluetooth and Bluetooth Low Energy. Used mainly for connectivity of wearable devices obtaining biophysical signals or indoor location systems.

Wireless system performance is conditioned mainly by receiver signal variation and observed interference levels. The main elements which must be considered are as follows:

a) **Antennas**: They transform guided waves into radiated waves and vice versa. Depending on their geometry and the materials employed, they can exhibit different values of gain and radiation diagrams.

b) **Receiver sensitivity**: Received signals are decoded, with minimum-power-level thresholds as a function of parameters such as transmission bit rate, modulation and coding scheme and hardware constraints. As a general rule, the higher the required transmission bit rate, the sensitivity threshold is more demanding, thus reducing the coverage level.

c) **Wireless channel**: It is the wireless path through which the signal follows from the transmitter to the receiver. As a function of different parameters, such as frequency of operation, distance or the structure of the surrounding environment, losses vary, which impacts on the maximum distance of operation for the communication links.

In order to analyse the deployment requirements of wireless communication systems and hence the feasibility of employing one class of system or another, it is necessary to obtain the maximum transmission link distance as a function of receiver sensitivity thresholds, which gives rise to coverage/capacity relations. In this way, a simplified analytical approach can be followed, given by the following expressions:

$$P_{RX} \geq SENS_{RX} \tag{9.1}$$

$$P_{RX} = P_{TX} - L_{(cable-feedTX)} + G_{(AntTX)} - L_{prop} + G_{(AntRX)} - L_{(cable-feedRX)} \tag{9.2}$$

where

- P_{RX}: Power level at receiver end of communication link in log scale.

- $SENS_{RX}$: Receiver sensitivity threshold, which depends on the parameters such as binary transmission rate, modulation and coding schemes and transceiver specifications (such as amplifier noise factors or device phase noise)

- P_{TX}: Transmission power level in log scale, which varies depending on parameters such as power control mechanisms and terminal class, among others.

- $L_{cable-feedTX} - L_{cable-feedRX}$: Losses corresponding to the transmission lines and cables employed for the feeding network, antenna matching circuits, power divider, power coupling and diplexer filters, at the transmitter/receiver side, respectively.

- $G_{AntTX} - G_{AntRX}$: Gain of transmitter/receiver antenna, which depends on the radiation diagram of the corresponding antenna element. Effects such as human body presence, which produces impedance mismatch, frequency shift and modification in radiation diagram, need to be considered.

- L_{prop}: Propagation losses, accounting the different physical phenomena related with the interaction of electromagnetic waves with the surrounding environment, as well as to inherent propagation mechanisms.

The highest variability and usually the most limiting factor in coverage/capacity relations is given by the propagation losses experienced by wireless links. The mechanisms that influence these losses are the following:

a) **Free space losses:** Exhibiting higher losses as the distance between transmitter and receiver increases, as well as frequency dependence.

b) **Atmospheric losses:** Given by the interaction of electromagnetic waves with gases as well as hydrometeors in the atmosphere (mainly at the troposphere level). Losses increase with frequency, particularly in the millimetre wave range, with different absorption peaks given by the presence of different gases such forms of H_2O, CO_X, NO_x or N_2, among others. In the case of IoMT applications, usually frequency bands in the sub 6 GHz range are considered, which exhibit low atmospheric losses. The future use of millimetre wave frequencies gives rise to short transmission ranges, especially in the case of considering human body interaction (owing to additional body losses, later described), which leads mainly to body area network applications.

c) **Interaction with material objects:** The presence of different elements in the wireless communication path derives into situations in which the propagating waves interact with these elements (e.g. furnishings, vegetation, presence of human bodies, etc.). This results in reflected, refracted, diffracted and scattered waves, being the main consequence of the increase in the losses experienced by the propagating electromagnetic waves, decreasing the effective coverage radius. The effect of these interactions is described by deriving the corresponding transmission and reflection coefficients by the application of Fresnel equations, which depend on the frequency, polarization, conductivity, dielectric constant and loss tangent of the different material elements within the scenarios under analysis. Diffraction losses are given by the presence of elements such as corners, edges or wedges, which by means of Huygens law re-radiates new diffracted wave fronts, which are strongly dependent on the shape and material of the diffraction region. This will be usually the case with the presence objects with sharp edges, such as building corners or in the case of indoor environments, furniture or infrastructure elements. Additionally, the presence of non-homogeneous and rough surfaces gives rise to diffuse scattering, in which besides the corresponding reflected wave, a set of randomly disposed reflected wave components of small amplitude is generated, leading to an effective decrease in the received power levels and hence reducing overall coverage. The main elements for diffuse scattering are given by building facades/walls and vegetation. There is also increased interest in the effect of diffused scattering caused by human body interaction, which is a variable to consider in the case of IoMT, particularly in the case of taking advantage of wearable transceivers.

d) **Human body presence:** IoMT applications are in many cases user-centric, making use of wearable devices in stand-alone or in a body area network configuration. Therefore, interaction of electromagnetic waves with the body of the users is unavoidable. The human body can be considered as an object present in the scenario under analysis in which wireless communication systems operate, requiring specific considerations [330,331]. On the one hand, the human body is composed of multiple tissues, with variable (but usually high) water content and different dielectric constant, loss tangent and conductivity values. This gives rise to losses in the case of intra-body propagation, as well as losses owing to off-body propagation mechanisms. The latter is also given by the fact that the presence of the human body (as well other elements, such as garments worn by the users) produces additional effects, such as changes in antenna impedance and variation in radiation diagram characteristics, which can limit the performance of wireless links. Other considerations must also be taken into account, such as the need for low-profile, ergonomic and conformable devices, which again limit the performance. Different approaches have been proposed for the integration of wireless transceivers in wearables, such as the use of flexible electronics (implemented with techniques such as inkjet or screen printing), miniaturized chip antennas or embedded conductive textiles, among others.

IoMT applications can span from social sensor network parameters to monitor user behaviour (e.g. presence sensors, accelerometers to monitor vertical/horizontal positions and hence emergency situations owing to falls, pressure sensor in beds, etc.), continuous monitoring of biophysical signals (e.g. ECG, EEG, EMG, temperature, oxygen saturation level, etc.), real-time transmission of audio/video signals for remote assistance or AR/VR information for medical diagnosis/training/procedures, just to name a few. These applications have different QoS/QoE parameters, with transmission bit rates in the range of 1 Kbps to over 1 Gbps or delay tolerance from 5 ms (e.g. remote robotic surgery) to several seconds (for device telemetry). On top of the application requirements, the impact of interference must also be considered, as this will degrade receiver performance. Interference sources can arise either from neighbouring users of our wireless communication system (intra-system interference), from other wireless communication systems (inter-system) or they can be generated by other external sources, such as brush motors, inductive arch welding, etc. [332,333]. Therefore, coverage/capacity analysis can provide insight in relation to the capabilities in network deployment as a function of the different available wireless communication systems. With this in mind, different results have been obtained and are presented in Figures 9.2, 9.3 and 9.4 related with coverage/capacity estimations, as a function of the employed frequency band and wireless system.

As it can be seen, depending on the frequency of operation, wireless system parameters and receiver sensitivity thresholds, communication link ranges can vary from metres to over several kilometres. It can be seen that if QoS parameters become more stringent, such as an increase in required transmission bit rate, in general coverage radius will decrease. Moreover, as interference values increase within the

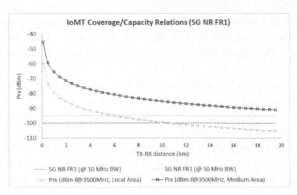

Figure 9.2 Estimation of coverage/capacity relations for LPWAN systems operating in 433 MHz, 868 MHz and 2.4 GHz

operating scenarios of the IoMT wireless systems, this will limit receiver performance (i.e. equivalent to degradation in receiver sensitivity value) which in turn will also reduce maximum wireless link distance. The values obtained consider in general line-of-sight conditions; therefore, if partial line-of-sight or non-line-of-sight conditions take place, expected coverage distances will be further reduced. Once that the impact of wireless channel behaviour in terms of coverage/capacity considerations has been described, we will now discuss the impact in communication system within IoMT applications given by interoperability, distributed computing resources and related security issues.

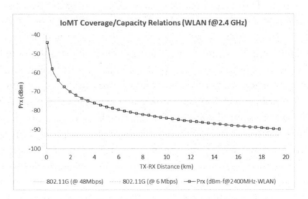

Figure 9.3 Estimation of coverage/capacity relations for 5G NR FR1 systems operating in 3.5 GHz

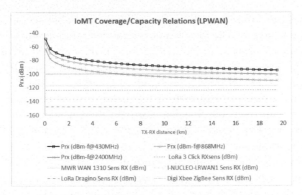

Figure 9.4 Estimation of coverage/capacity relations for WLAN (f@2.4 GHz) systems, considering urban scenarios in predominant LOS link conditions

9.2 DATA STANDARDIZATION AND INTEROPERABILITY IN IOMT ARCHITECTURES

Data governance and management is crucial for ensuring data quality in current and future IoT and IoMT frameworks. In this context, interoperability and standardization are regarded as strategic enablers for versatile, seamless integration. The state of affairs of the information and communication technologies (ICT) in the healthcare environment includes a gradually rising number of government policies and initiatives as well as a wide variety of standardization bodies and entities. In this subsection, an in-depth overview of the most relevant actors, organizations, standards and norms related to IoT and, particularly, IoMT is described. Although platitudinous enough, IoT solutions, as inherently conveyed by the 'I' in the acronym, are based on the internet. Therefore, web and internet communication standards are the core foundation on which IoT and IoMT systems are built. There is a broad range of efforts related to IoT, ranging from physical protocols, such as Bluetooth Low Energy (BLE) or Narrow Band IoT (NB-IoT), to higher level formats, such as JavaScript Object Notation (JSON). In this group of internet-related protocols, we could include several recent IoT protocols, designed to deliver lightweight machine-to-machine communications. Examples thereof are the Constrained Application Protocol (CoAP) [333], the Message Queuing Telemetry Transport (MQTT), the Advanced Message Queuing Protocol (AMQP), or the Data Distribution Service (DDS).

A number of organizations work towards the development of novel and comprehensive norms expected to pave the way for enhanced interoperability. A Standards Development Organization (SDO) is an entity whose prime activity is to define, coordinate and/or promote consensus standards relevant for the related industry. In fact, they are usually proposed by the very stakeholders, in need for a formal stability within their domain. At the moment of writing, the principal organizations coordinating the development of medical informatics standards, applicable to IoMT scenarios, are presented as follows. The International Organization for Standardization (ISO) is a body for defining international standards. However, ISO also publishes technical reports, technical specifications, publicly available specifications, technical corrigenda and guides. The European Committee for Standardization (CEN, from French 'Committee European of Normalization') is the foremost organization in this field located in Europe. Moreover, in every country, there is usually a national organization acting as a CEN mirror, in charge of coordinating the national activities. For example, in the case of Spain (where the authors of this book chapter are from), the national CEN mirror is the Spanish Normalization Association (AENOR, from Spanish 'Asociación Española de Normalización y Certificación'). There are different subgroups working on standardization in the field of Health ICT. The most pertinent ones for this field are Technical Committee 251 (CEN/TC 251) and Technical Committee 139 (AEN/CTN 139), respectively. At a technical level, the Institute of Electrical and Electronics Engineers (IEEE) is an international non-for-profit association engaged with standards development at a wide scope, including electrical and electronic engineering, telecommunications, informatics, cyber security and health, among others.

Diving more specifically into the healthcare context, a number of standards development organizations are active in this field For example, Health Level Seven (HL7) International, which is a well-known developer of health data interoperability standards or Integrating the Healthcare Enterprise (IHE), is an organization that leverages health interoperability standards to propose profiles for improved health data governance. Continua Health Alliance, now part of the Personal Connected Health Alliance (PCHA), was created by various stakeholders (that is to say, academia, healthcare professionals, medical device manufacturers and technology firms) to encourage the coordinated use of these standards. The PCHA is a membership-based company of the Healthcare Information and Management Systems Society (HIMSS), an organization aimed at enhancing the quality and access to healthcare by means of an adequate use of information technology and health management systems.

IEEE, while aiming at a broader scope, is also dedicating ongoing effort to defining IoT standards. Among the various initiatives, we could emphasize the following four, since they are closely related to IoT and, therefore, to IoMT scenarios. First, the IEEE 2413-2019 is a document that promotes a standardized architectural framework for IoT. Such architecture framework description is driven by concerns usually shared by stakeholders of IoT systems across multiple domains. In this document, an abstract foundation for the notion of 'things' in the IoT is provided. It also elaborates a compendium of architecture viewpoints stemmed from the shared concerns mentioned above in order to create the core of the framework described in this document. Second, the IEEE P2510 copes with sensors, which are crucial for an IoT ecosystem. More specifically, it aims at establishing quality of data sensor parameters in the IoT environment. This document therefore provides a shared framework for sensor-related issues (such as units, terminology, limits, etc.). Third, the IEEE P1451-99 is a document devoted to the harmonization and security of IoT devices and systems. This standard aims at defining a way for sharing data, taking into account the interoperability and security of the messages over the network, independently of the specific communication technology underneath. The backend would be based on the eXtensible Messaging and Presence Protocol (XMPP), thus providing features such as globally authenticated identities, authorization, presence, life cycle management, interoperable communication, IoT discovery and provisioning; finally, the IEEE P2733, which promotes IoT data and device interoperability, but enforcing Trust, Identity, Privacy, Protection, Safety, Security (TIPPSS). The main purpose is to enable secured data sharing in connected healthcare while protecting patient privacy and security. Within the IoT field, there are multiple domains, such as smart manufacturing, industry 4.0, smart grid, smart cities or smart logistics, to name only a few. One of the most complex scenarios is arguably the smart healthcare domain, due to the intricate data models inherent to this context. Some of the first to arrive were the terminologies, such as the Systematized Nomenclature of Medicine (SNOMED) or Logical Observation Identifiers Names and Codes (LOINC), whose main aim is to provide a reliable, comprehensive way to index and identify all health-related terms there exist. On top of that, sophisticated protocols appear, such as the CEN/ISO 13606 standard or the openEHR norm, both initiatives devoted to the interoperable exchange of electronic health records (EHRs). The main objective of the CEN/ISO 13606 standard is to define a detailed and stable information architecture for communicating part or all of EHRs of a patient between different EHR systems, or between an EHR system and other health information systems (HIS). openEHR is a compound of open specifications, clinical models and software aimed to create medical standards and build interoperable information solutions in the healthcare domain. CEN/ISO 13606 and openEHR share a common objective and structure. Indeed, the fundamental shareable specifications of clinical information (called archetypes) could be mutually transcoded. A simpler, more lightweight approach was established by version 4 of the HL7 standard, commonly referred to as Fast Healthcare Interoperability Resources (FHIR). This standard provides an Hypertext Transfer Protocol (HTTP)-based RESTful Application Programing Interface (API) for interoperable health data exchange. Related to all these are the ontologies, which provide formal representation of shared concepts and the relationships among them within the medical domain. In this context, a noteworthy initiative is ISO/IEEE 11073, a standard for medical device interoperability that has been evolving throughout the last years. First, it aimed at the Point of Care (PoC), that is typically bigger devices close to hospital beds. In parallel, the nomenclature was defined by means of the IEEE 11073-10101 document. Second, it evolved towards Personal Health Devices (PHDs), covering smaller medical devices in home scenarios with a local manager capable of handling all of them simultaneously. The core document of this version of the standard was the ISO/IEEE 11073-20601, referred to as the optimized exchange protocol. This document defined a Domain Information Model (DIM), a service model and a communication model. The PHD version also defined several device specialization profiles (ISO/IEEE 11073-104zz), one for each sensor to be modelled, e.g. the pulse oximeter (ISO/IEEE 11073-10404),the blood pressure monitor (ISO/IEEE 11073-10407) or the electrocardiogram (ISO/IEEE 11073-10406). Along with that, the Continua Health Alliance proposed design and implementation guidelines to promote the global adoption of this standard. However, such guidelines, despite continuous improvement, have had relative success so far. The main concerns are the inevitability of defining and implementing one profile per device type, the complexity of sending measurements directly to the cloud and the limited (albeit feasible) transcoding to HL7 FHIR, which arguably is the reference standard in current mobile health applications. Thus, in order to overcome these issues, a new Abstract COntent Model (ACOM) for PHDs is currently under development, with reference name project IEEE P11073-10206 [334]. It aims at defining an abstract model for devices based on the DIM and nomenclature previously defined for PHDs. The main advantages would be the straightforward binary representation of HL7 FHIR resources, the possibility of deploying direct-to-cloud architectures (there is an ongoing effort by IHE and PCHA) and the definition of a generic health sensor model for all types of sensors (being currently developed by the Bluetooth special interest group), simplifying thereby the implementation of scenarios with multiple sensors. A structured table summarizing all related acronyms of this subsection is provided in Table 9.2.

9.2.1 INCORPORATION OF DATA STANDARDIZATION IN IOMT ARCHITECTURES

The incorporation of IoT and IoMT standards to IoMT architectures provides several advantages and disadvantages. Among the advantages, we could name the following. First, it would provide enhanced interoperability and integration among the different healthcare actors involved. Second, the extract, transform and load (ETL) operations would become simpler, since they operate consistently, even though when incorporating new devices to the ecosystem. Third, the definition of precise health data models opens the door to effective reasoning over the data, which could help to find patients at risk by means of software algorithms or artificial intelligence. Fourth, it would make it easier for individuals to become co-producers of health, since the medical data could be straightforwardly sent and integrated to EHRs. Fifth, this also would benefit patients, who would be able to access, download and inspect (with open-source software applications) their own data, typically stored today at the hospital servers, often unavailable to patients. Finally, the healthcare information systems (HIS) of the hospitals would become easier to develop and maintain. On the other hand, there are some disadvantages to the standardization of IoMT architectures. First, the standardization arena is rather fragmented, moreover taking into account that this section provides a rather comprehensive but incomplete overview, limited to the most relevant efforts. This situation is problematic for developers, architects and health information systems managers. Second, some standards are excessively complex to implement, which hurdles wider adoption. Third, there is a cost attached to the incorporation of standards to the devices or architectures, in several terms, such as economic, temporal and/or human resources terms. This naturally increments the price of the solution at the end. Finally, there is also an additional information-related cost, in terms of memory and computing time, which directly affects the battery life, critical in IoMT devices. As a result, the interoperability and standardization arena in IoMT is a complex environment. A plethora of IoT and IoMT formats, protocols and standards have been proposed, but the seamless application thereof to IoMT ecosystems requires further research. In general, as a

Table 9.2

Acronyms Related to Data Standardization and Interoperability in IoMT Architectures

Acronym	Stands for
GENERIC INTERNET-RELATED ACRONYMS	
ICT	Information and Communication Technologies
IoT	Internet of Things
IoMT	Internet of Medical Things
HTTP	Hypertext Transfer Protocol
API	Application Programing Interface
TIPPSS	Trust, Identity, Privacy, Protection, Safety, Security
ETL	Extract, Transform and Load
GENERIC IoT-RELATED PROTOCOLS	
BLE	Bluetooth Low Energy
NB-IoT	Narrow Band IoT
JSON	JavaScript Object Notation
XMPP	eXtensible Messaging and Presence Protocol
CoAP	Constrained Application Protocol
MQTT	Message Queuing Telemetry Transport
AMQP	Advanced Message Queuing Protocol
DDS	Data Distribution Service
TECHNICAL ORGANIZATIONS	
SDO	Standards Development Organization
ISO	The International Organization for Standardization
CEN	European Committee for Standardization
AENOR	Spanish Normalization Association
IEEE	Institute of Electrical and Electronics Engineers
TECHNICAL ORGANIZATIONS IN THE MEDICAL DOMAIN	
HL7	Health Level Seven
IHE	Integrating the Healthcare Enterprise
PCHA	Personal Connected Health Alliance
HIMSS	Healthcare Information and Management Systems Society
MEDICAL-RELATED STANDARDIZATION ACRONYMS	
SNOMED	Systematized Nomenclature of Medicine
LOINC	Logical Observation Identifiers Names and Codes
FHIR	Fast Healthcare Interoperability Resources
EHR	Electronic Health Records
HIS	Health Information Systems
PoC	Point of Care
PHD	Personal Health Devices

final reflection on this matter, the incorporation of standards to IoMT architectures poses a delicate trade-off between advanced interoperability and different costs.

9.3 DISTRIBUTED AND CLOUD COMPUTING CAPABILITIES

An IoHT system needs, as any other information system does, to collect, process, store, share and present information. In this case, the information to be handled has some special features that must be taken into account. The information reflects patients' medical data, which is protected by different regulations (in the case of the European Union by the GPDR) and must be treated in a special way. This implies a need for encryption and anonymization of the information, so that the information is unbundled from any data that would allow a third party to find out to which patient the information corresponds. This can be done by hash functions, by temporary identifiers that expire in short periods of time, or other solutions or combinations of them. IoT devices send patient's information to an aggregator node (fog) located in the patient's immediate environment (patient's home) to which they are univocally linked via wireless networks (BLE or similar). This minimizes the risk of compromising patient information, as the aggregator takes care of the proper encryption of the information before it is sent to the information system located in the cloud. Furthermore, it reduces the communication latency. This secure transmission will guarantee both the integrity of the messages and the authenticity of the sender and receiver. The aggregator is responsible for negotiating with the information system the management of temporary identifiers and the encryption mechanism. Figure 9.5 shows a classical schema of computing and storage organization with three layers: edge, fog and cloud layers. IoT devices are located at the edge layer and have a limited capacity of both computing and storage. At the fog layer, aggregators have greater computing, storage and communication capacity. This ensures a secure communication with the next level and, in case of communication interruption, allows

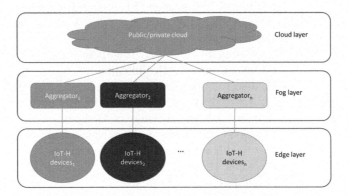

Figure 9.5 A classical schema of computing and storage organization: edge, fog and cloud layers.

the temporary storage of the information collected by the IoT network until it can be transmitted to the cloud level. Finally, the cloud layer hosts the HIS. This cloud may be either a public or a private solution according to the privacy and security requirements of each organization, or even a hybrid solution. When greater control of information is required and sufficient resources are available, a private cloud is often chosen over the alternative of a public cloud, which requires fewer resources on the part of the organization, but implies less control over the data.

Healthcare IoT cloud-based proposals are neither new nor novel [335, 336], although new proposals for patient (with chronical diseases) monitoring using narrowband IoT technologies are currently being put forward [337, 338]. The main drawback of these technologies is the latency introduced, which makes them unsuitable for real-time monitoring of vital signs. This is further aggravated when IoT devices communicate directly over a cloud-based information system, without using an edge/fog solution. Security is a key aspect, so both patient anonymity and communication encryption must be guaranteed but, in addition, the information must also be stored dissociated from any data that could allow an unauthorized identification of the patient, regardless of the computing and storage architecture chosen (cloud/fog/edge). Many proposals have addressed these issues, as [339, 340], and there are sure to be more proposals that will continue to be formulated, since these are issues that have not yet been solved.

Data exchange between IoT monitoring devices and the information system is also a relevant issue to be considered. Different markup languages as XML and JSON (or even YAML) can be considered, as occurs with FHIR, so HIS should natively support both interchange formats. HIS, either because they directly implement HL7 or because they use service buses to implement data ingestion from the IoT networks, must deal with XML/JSON messages. NextGen Connect (previously known as Mirt Connect) is an example of a service bus, a cross-platform interface engine used to grant bi-directional sending/receiving of many types of messages, in this case to ensure the semantic interoperability of the data collected with the HL7 messaging standard. HIS implementations may concern a unique instance, but this is not the norm. For reasons of redundancy, but also of scalability, cloud solutions that leverage hyperconverged solutions are often used by the providers of these solutions. In this scenario, data ingestion from IoT devices is often performed at the aggregators side, which communicate directly by means of HL7 messages with the HIS hosted at the cloud side. The use of some elements of HL7 as Clinical Document Architecture (CDA), Continuity of Care Record (CCR), Continuity of Care Document (CCD) and Consolidated Clinical Document Architecture (CCDA) allows an easy customization of any HIS system to the corresponding language, which is an important aspect when opting for cloud-based systems. This is especially important when the same HIS must support interaction in different languages, or when the same provider supports different customers. The latter case is particularly sensitive when it comes to ensuring the protection of medical record data. Opting for cloud solutions (public or private) helps to reduce HIS implementation and operating costs [341–346], mainly due to the dynamic scalability provided by virtualization. Performing system snapshots is really simple and fast, allowing for quick and efficient system recovery in case of failure. From the point of view of system integration, the use of archetypes and ontologies greatly facilitates the interoperability of HIS with legacy systems. This is possible through cloud systems by publishing web services or by using programming APIs. In any case, it is an issue to be considered by those responsible for healthcare management.

Currently, these systems are betting heavily on the ability to learn and recognize patterns [347–351]. This implies the use of machine learning techniques, for which it is not only necessary to have adequate computing capabilities like GPU, but it is just as important, if not more, to have enough learning samples to make such learning possible. In such context, the use of informed machine learning [352] by integrating prior knowledge into the training process may aid to avoid this issue. However, the biggest evolution in this field seems to come from digital twins (DTs). Some authors, as [353], consider that DT technology 'has the potential to transform healthcare in a variety of ways – improving the diagnosis and treatment of patients, streamlining preventative care and facilitating new approaches for hospital planning'. DTs seem to be pervasively used to digitalize any assets of a health organization [354, 355], but they will also be used to provide personalized medicine [356–358], to reproduce patients' previous pathologies before surgery, and even more. A DT of any vital organ may represent the physical behaviour (electrical, mechanical, biochemical...). This allows not only to know the behaviour of this organ in the patient, but also to study the best way to address their pathologies both at the surgical level and at any other level. In this context, the ability to use DT technology to reconstruct all or part of a patient's organs in order to provide real and effective personalized medicine will be crucial. This can be done with on premise proprietary solutions developed specifically for each hospital or even as a service (Digital Twin as a Service, DTaaS).

9.4   SECURITY

The IoMT is already shaping healthcare with significant benefits for patients, clinicians and medical device providers. The emergence of new and additional connectivity technologies in IoMT is enabling more and better remote collection and transmission of data from users and their environments. At the same time, such connectivity is considered a risk from a cyber security point of view. Nowadays, cyberattacks are a complex, constantly evolving global threat. Cyber security vulnerabilities can emerge in any medical device that can be connected to another electronic device or network, disrupting its function and compromising the data security. In addition, vulnerable medical devices may be harnessed as part of a botnet to launch attacks on other targets; as a back channel to breach the security of hospital or clinic networks; to extract ransoms; to harm a patient or user of the device and to inflict other financial or reputational damages onto device manufacturers, clinics and patients [359, 360].It is worth highlighting that in healthcare services and environments, privacy of personal data in transit (e.g. managed on a healthcare cloud, transmitted across networks, etc.) needs to offer a high level of assurance. Furthermore, confidentiality and integrity of data is of utmost importance, so emphasis should also be placed on data storage and processing. With a large number of IoMT devices on the rise in the healthcare ecosystem, the need for strong security measures is essential. Two complementary strategies are presented below, with the aim of guaranteeing the security of IoMT devices and their compliance with current standards in the field of cyber security and medical devices development: IEC 62443, IEC 62304 and ISO 13485.

9.4.1 RISK-BASED CYBER SECURITY MANAGEMENT

The first step in the process is to develop a holistic risk-based cyber security plan that addresses overall vulnerability issues related to safety, security, privacy, software and design. Within this plan, medical device manufacturers should make provisions to ensure that device design will be simple and easy to update, while adhering to regulatory best practices. Moreover, manufacturers should plan vulnerability management processes to ensure that fixes can be rapidly developed and deployed to their products. At the same time, they will need to define processes and protocols to handle security breaches that could arise with the setup and maintenance of IoMT devices. In IEC 62443 standard, risk is defined as the result of the following equation:

$$Risk = Threat \times Vulnerability \times Consequence \qquad (9.3)$$

Considering the following:

- *Threat*: Potential for violation of security, which exists when there is a circumstance, capability, action or event that could breach security and cause harm

- *Vulnerability*: Flaw or weakness in a system's design, implementation or operation and management that could be exploited to violate the system's integrity or security policy

- *Consequences*: Flaw or weakness in a system's design, implementation or operation and management that could be exploited to violate the system's integrity or security policy

According to IEC 62443 standard, cyber-security-related risks should be identified and classified and mitigation actions should be defined in order to achieve desired security levels. This methodical approach allows device hardening to improve their ability withstand a cyberattack. Table 9.3 summarizes security level (SL) coupled with the type of attacker.

In order to empower the use of IoT in the medical healthcare domain, it is necessary to recognize and examine specific qualities of IoMT including security requirements, vulnerabilities and countermeasures, as well as their implications from the healthcare perspective. A good risk assessment should provide a risk profile, highest severity consequence threats, vulnerabilities leading to the highest risks and target SLs for the assessed devices. Table 9.4 shows typical attacks in terms of effects and mitigation actions [361–363]. Some actions apply on the device and others in the service architecture.

Table 9.3
Security Levels Defined in IEC 62443

Security Level	Target	Skills	Motivations	Means	Resources
SL1	Casual or coincidental	Violations	No attack skills	Mistakes	Non-intentional individual
SL2	Cybercrime hacker	Generic	Low	Simple	Low (isolated individual)
SL3	Hacktivist and terrorist	Specific	Moderate	Sophisticated (attack)	Moderate (hacker group)
SL4	Nation	State	Specific	High sophisticated (campaign)	Extended (multidisciplinary teams)

9.4.2 SECURITY BY DESIGN

Countering cyberattacks starts by incorporating secure measures from the beginning of a device or app development, to mitigate threats. Security is a crucial objective at all stages of product creation and deployment. It addresses the challenge that, in many historic hardware deployments and instances of IoT design, security considerations were often included late in the design and prototyping phase, provoking serious security breaches. Security by design is a methodology that ensures security and privacy by design and by default. Accordingly, an effective and proactive means to reduce the number and severity of vulnerabilities in IoT is to develop applications in a secure manner, making use of secure Software Development Life Cycle (sSDLC) principles and developers trained in secure coding. Several security challenges of the

Table 9.4
Typical Attacks in Smart Health

Attack	Effect	Mitigation
Denial of Service (DoS)	Distributed attack affects availability of system services	Early intrusion detection
Routing Attack	Change route information	Continuous route monitoring
Sensor Attack	Data modification	Node failure and replacement detection
Replay Attack	Drop data packets	Data freshness techniques

IoT can be addressed by establishing a set of secure development guidelines, such as checking for security vulnerabilities, secure deployment, ensuring continuity of secure development in cases of integrators, continuous delivery, etc. Several security challenges of the IoMT can be addressed by establishing a set of specific security considerations and guidelines to be taken into account during IoMT's entire development life cycle. One of the SDLC is shown in Figure 9.6.

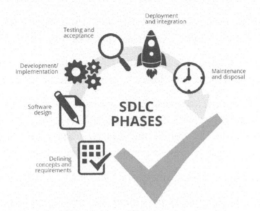

Figure 9.6   Secure SDLC [329]

9.5   CONSIDERATIONS FOR AN IOMT-DEPLOYED USE CASE

Patient-centred use cases for the provision of health services based on IoMT can be found in each of the medical scenarios. In the case of public health systems such as in Spain, the greatest efficiency of the system is found in patients with chronic diseases, such as diabetes, high blood pressure, respiratory failure, asthma, etc. Also of great interest are use cases based on screening of patients with asymptomatic pathologies such as cancer (breast, colon, etc.) as well as other pathologies such as those associated with diabetes, ageing, etc. In short, there are many fronts in innovation that can be done both at a technological level, such as human resources (new professions) and management of health processes, etc. An innovation that must be carried out from a holistic point of view and not just only technological. In our closest environment, both screening strategies and clinical trials spin around patients as home hospitalization of mild or moderate COVID-19 patients, generally asymptomatic, fundus screening, etc., has been addressed [364]. Without going into depth on the deployment of these health services based on IoMT describing in detail the medical devices and communications used, standardization and security, as well as the processing of the data itself, aspects that have been valued in other parts of this chapter, it seems appropriate to describe briefly those aspects that arise from the deployment itself. One example for a practical case study is given by eye fundus screening. The prevalence of diabetic patients can be around 10% in first world countries; as an example, in the region of Navarra, Spain, around 7%, approx. 50,000 patients, according to annual reports. Given these figures, a fundus screening strategy in order to prevent retinal pathologies such as RD, AMD, etc., is compulsory. The implementation of an eye fundus diagnosis and monitoring system is feasible following the IoMT paradigms. The necessary technology integrates the following elements:

- *Non-Mydriatic Fundus Camera* with mobility, with internet connection (wired or wireless) and with medical image transmission standards such as DICOM

- Hospital information systems (HIS) including appointment management (RIS), worklist management, electronic prescription, EHR, PACS servers, etc.

- Mature artificial intelligence algorithms for medical image processing with a very high sensitivity and specificity in order not to generate long waiting lists.

- *Other support elements*: Customized mobility for transport (vans, small lorries, etc.) including the medical devices needed (non-mydriatic fundus camera, OCT, tonometer, etc.) as well as the necessary stays for patients. Likewise, it should have high-speed wireless communication, servers, etc.

In relation to the necessary professionals, the following can be distinguished:

- Non-sanitary or basic sanitary personnel (van drivers), who could have the necessary skills to handle the non-mydriatic fundus camera, take the photographs, as well as their subsequent transmission to the PACS, always with close collaboration with the healthcare personnel, could manage the patients appropriately.

- Physicians specialized in ophthalmology, who are mainly responsible for the operation of the service, as well as for making decisions about the pathology, medical prescription, etc. In short, the main actors of this strategy.

The successful integration of this eye funds diagnosis and analysis systems requires the definition and implementation of a process model that can be included within the general hospital complex procedures. In this case, the process model considers the following stages:

a) Patients are regularly cited, based on current medical evidence and in accordance with the evolution of medical knowledge. This appointment management is carried out automatically using the HIS and with the appropriate periodicity, always based on the medical evidence of the moment.

b) Patient centric: Where are patients cited? Based on the public health system in Spain, patients are cited at their local health centre or its area of influence where the necessary room is available for an adequate location of mobility to carry out the tests, as well as for the usual waiting of the patient.

c) The mobility device (van or small lorries) equipped with the necessary medical and communication technology travels to the health centres where the patients have been cited. These trips must be based on good route management using current technologies in order to minimize distance and maximize the number of daily or weekly patients cited depending on the needs of the system.

From a technological point of view, the technology is mature (HIS, medical devices, communications, apps, AI algorithms for both signal and image processing, maps, etc.) and it is working perfectly, sometimes in isolation, but it may be a good time for its integration. From a human resources point of view, the rise of other types of multidisciplinary professions (drivers, non-specialized health personnel, biomedical engineers, etc.) could also be positive. The so-called digitization of health services entails this multidisciplinary approach between different fields of knowledge and new professions. The problems could come from the regulatory point of view, but it is true that there is an evolution towards patient-centred health services, so these initiatives that seek efficiency in the management of resources should always be valued public, as well as in the adequate provision of health services. It is not difficult to imagine that this redesign could be used to include another type of IoMT technology for the provision of other health services (electrocardiography, echocardiography, etc.) in a way that makes intensive and efficient use of the said technology, for the sake of system efficiency and thinking about the provision of patient-centred digital health services.

10 An Energy-Efficient Data Routing and Aggregation Protocol for WBANs

Roopali Punj and Rakesh Kumar

CONTENTS

10.1 INTRODUCTION

The rapid cost-effective research in the field of wireless sensor technologies, wearable devices and IoT has revolutionized the way to deal with chronic diseases, obesity, cardiovascular diseases, diabetes and problems of ageing population. Sensor nodes, wearable or implanted, both continuously monitor the patient forming Wireless Body Area Networks (WBANs) as each sensor node is able to sense, communicate and process [365]. Sensor nodes can sense various physiological parameters and then transmit to the medical server. The data on server is accessible to the patient as well as to the doctor for further analysis and diagnosis as shown in Figure 10.1 [366, 367]. The modern-day healthcare systems are better than conventional healthcare systems as they are able to detect diseases and their symptoms at early stages. WBANs can allow patient to be at home while being monitored by medical fraternity. This reduces hospital costs and improves the quality of life [368]. However, several challenging issues such as energy consumption, network lifetime, Specific Absorption Rate (SAR), interference, fault tolerance, propagation delay and dynamic data and network topologies hinder the widespread usage of WBANs for health and activity monitoring [369].

DOI: 10.1201/9781003239895-10

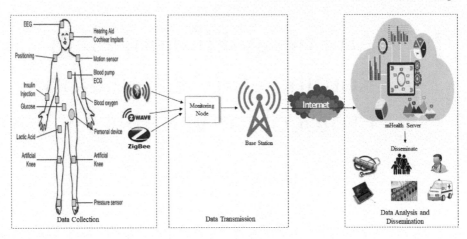

Figure 10.1   Wireless Body Area Networks [366]

The communication process consumes most of the energy, and it is difficult for sensor nodes to recharge or replace their batteries. As the sensor nodes sense continuously, transmitted data may be redundant. However, clustering the nodes and aggregating the data can save energy to some extent [370] by decreasing the network congestion, whereas aggregation is combining the data, collected from different sources. For instance, mathematical functions like maximum, minimum, average and concatenate can be used to aggregate data and can help in optimizing energy consumption, network lifetime and transmission cost [371, 372] without affecting the gathered measures.

In this chapter, we propose an efficient data routing and aggregation scheme that dynamically creates clusters in the network. Cluster head (CH), which is a node similar to other nodes in the network with maximal energy at that particular instance, receives continuous data from the nodes and transmit to the intermediary node, which performs aggregation, on the basis of variance and data priority. The effectiveness of the proposed protocol is shown by promising results that imply exclusive performance to route and aggregate the data, hence improving energy consumption and network lifetime.

The significance of the proposed data routing technique is that for the purpose of clustering, CHs are selected dynamically and clusters are formed in such a way that they are not widely dispersed. This helps in balancing load at cluster members as well as at the CH. Also, in order to reduce the network congestion, redundant data is concatenated based on variance, priority and time stamp of the data packet.

10.1.1   RELATED WORK

In this section, we present a concise discussion about various state-of-the-art techniques for WBANs based on routing and aggregation proposed by various researchers to bring deeper insight into ubiquitous healthcare applications.

In [373], the author presented a review of data fusion techniques providing a classification of data aggregation techniques. The author explained existing techniques and methods for data association, state estimation and decision fusion along with their mathematical explanations along with wide range of application domains where various data fusion techniques could be applied. The author reviewed the most relevant studies available for data fusion on the basis of computational cost and delay in the communication.

In [374], the authors have proposed a data aggregation scheme that forwards data as per different priorities set for data. The proposed protocol has better performance measures as it optimizes average delay, communication cost and packet delivery ratio. However, data security is not considered.

In [375], the authors proposed a multi-source framework for improving efficiency and scalability in prioritizing patients remotely. The authors focused on classification and prioritizing patients in health monitoring system and had improved accuracy. The proposed model was scalable in nature as it could accommodate all user requests. The proposed framework focused on the usage of data fusion in wireless healthcare applications. The simulation results had shown the improved accuracy of the proposed framework but there was a trade-off between the increasing number of users and system complexity. Also, the authors had not tested the framework on the real-time application.

In [376], authors proposed an efficient data aggregation technique that performs aggregation firstly at the node level and then at CH level. The technique is successful in reducing the number of data measures sent to the sink node. However, the aggregation process takes place at sensor nodes which consumes energy.

In [377], the authors proposed an optimized cost-effective routing protocol (OCER). It uses Genetic Algorithm for optimal route selection between source and sink for data transfer. It optimizes energy consumption and network lifetime. In [378], mobility and priority-based routing protocol for WBANs is proposed by the authors. The distance between source and sink varies while the patient is moving. These data priorities depend variation in mobility and on the condition of a patient. Forwarding just the critical data to sink optimizes resource utilization.

In [379], the authors presented a healthcare data aggregation scheme that uses peer-to-peer communication between sensor and aggregator nodes to share encrypted data. Then the aggregator node shares data with the next aggregator node or FoG server whichever is nearer. The node may not directly transmit data to the FOG server, so it encrypts its data and transmits it to the neighbouring aggregator node which in turn appends its encrypted data and transmits it to the FoG server. The major functionality of FoG server is of decrypting data and storing at cloud repositories. However, the basic WBAN parameters like residual energy and energy consumption are not taken care of.

In [380], the authors discuss the prevailing data aggregation issues focusing on propagation delay, energy utilization, data redundancy and accuracy and traffic load. In the presented model, the sensor node first sense the data and transmit it to the CH. Firstly, CH performs data aggregation but does not completely remove the redundant data. Then the CH transmits data to a storage node which is considered to have maximum residual energy. Secondly, the storage node performs data aggregation and completely removes the redundant data. It then transmits data to the base station. Therefore, it manages trade-off between energy efficiency and accuracy. As there is multi-level data aggregation in the proposed model, it reduces network lifetime.

In [381], the authors have proposed data aggregation and channelization framework where data is transmitted by selecting a cloud gateway for healthcare in post-disaster scenario. The Local Data Processing Units (LDPUs) perform aggregation and transmit data to the health cloud.

10.1.2 PROBLEM FORMULATION

In this section, we elaborate the proposed data aggregation technique and the subsequent sub-sections explain the methodology and implementation details for the proposed technique. The proposed technique focuses on aggregating the same or redundant data packets received from the same source at different time stamps which help in improving the network lifetime by reducing the total number of packets transmitted. The proposed data aggregation technique is elaborated which cost-effectively forwards the data. Sensor nodes consume most of their energy during data communication as compared to data acquisition and data processing [382]. Energy expenditure is calculated using Equation (10.1) at the transmitter end and Equation (10.2) at the receiving end, respectively, based on First-Order Radio model [383, 384].

$$E_{Tx}(p, r) = E_{elec} * r + \varepsilon_{Amp} * r * p^2 \tag{10.1}$$

$$E_{Rx}(r) = E_{elec} * r \tag{10.2}$$

where E_{Tx} and E_{Rx} represent energy consumption at transmitting and receiving end, respectively (sum of energy consumption of all electronic devices used at each end), E_{Telec} and E_{Relec} represent energy consumption by transmitter and receiver, respectively, and E_{Amp} represents energy consumption by amplifier for transmitting r-bit long message at p distance.

10.1.3 PROPOSED METHODOLOGY

The proposed scheme uses divide and conquer, the difference in variance and data priority for aggregating the data. The working of the proposed scheme is shown in Figure 10.2. It uses temporal correlation of data to reduce redundancy and helps in reducing the number of transmissions from source to sink required to complete the communication process.

10.1.4 CLUSTER FORMATION

Cluster formation avoids direct communication from source to sink as it is energy extensive. Each sensor node in the network is associated with its respective ID, energy levels and placed location. CH is the node with highest level of remaining energy. As CHs also have the same power and communicational abilities, an equal number of nodes is added to every cluster in order to achieve load balancing at the CH. The whole network can be covered by total clusters $CL = N/n$ where N is the total population and n is user-defined cluster members. Further, it is assumed that the CH is of the same communicational power as sensor nodes so data aggregation is not performed at CH. In order to balance load at the CH, sensor nodes transmit data to CH which in turn transmits it to the aggregator nodes. From the aggregator node, data is transmitted to the sink. A detailed description of other phases, namely, cluster setup phase, fitness evaluation and routing path selection is given in [370].

10.1.5 DATA AGGREGATION

At the aggregator node, data is received from the CH which in turn receives data packets from nodes in a cluster. As it receives collective data packets, it is necessary to reduce the packets into single units in order to calculate the difference in information contained in two packets from the same source. d_s^t is one data packet at sensor node s collected at time stamp t. Therefore, data received at CH from all cluster members is represented as $(d_1^1, d_1^2, d_1^3 \cdots d_1^n), (d_2^1, d_2^2, d_2^3 \cdots d_2^n), \cdots, (d_k^1, d_k^2, d_k^3 \cdots d_k^n)$. Next, D_s^{ch} is data received at the aggregator node from the CH ch and the sensor node s. Then this collective information received at the aggregator node needs to be extracted in order to discard redundant information. This process of data reduction is given in algorithm 1.

$$Diff(d_1^1, d_1^2) = \begin{cases} 1, & \text{if } |d_1^1 - d_1^2| \leq \delta \\ 0, & \text{otherwise} \end{cases} \tag{10.3}$$

$$Var_i = \frac{(d_i - \mu)^2}{l} \tag{10.4}$$

Algorithm 1 Data Reduction

Input: Data packets from CH received at FN_i
Output: Unit Data Packets

1: **if** $(n > i)$ **then**
2:    $M \leftarrow (i+n)/2$;
3: **end if**
4: DataReduction (D_{si}^{CHi}, M);
5: DataReduction $(M+1, D_{si}^{CHn})$;
6: $N \leftarrow$ total packets at FN_i
7: **for** $\forall N$ **do**
8:    DataAggregate$(N_1, N_2, ..., N_k)$;
9: **end for**

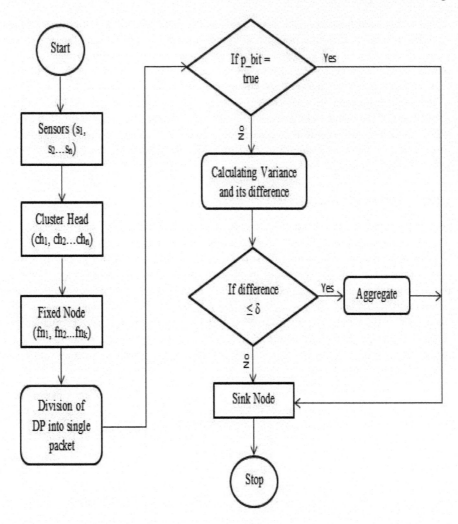

Figure 10.2   General framework for the proposed system

For all the single data packets extracted at the aggregator node, it checks if the priority bit is set or not. If the priority bit in data packet is true, then data is not aggregated as it contains critical information which needs to be transmitted to sink node on a priority basis without any delay. If the priority bit is not set, then k-means is applied on all data packets forming clusters equal to the actual number of clusters. Now each cluster has data packets with similar values. This helps us in calculating variance of the data packets from same source in each cluster using Equation (10.4) where d_i represents data, μ is mean value of all data packets and l is length of data packets from source i. The difference in variance of packets in different clusters received from the same source is calculated using Equation (10.3). If the difference is less than a set threshold δ, then data are aggregated based on their similarity index. Threshold level decides what level of similarity is accommodated in the process of aggregation and is selected as observed from the literature. Since we are considering health data, therefore, normal range of the physiological parameters is considered as threshold. The best representative of the information is selected and transmitted to the sink node. Otherwise, data packets contain dissimilar information and should not be aggregated. This process is explained in algorithm 2. The proposed technique contributes to decreasing redundant data and communication costs by decreasing the number of transmissions and re-transmissions while maintaining accuracy.

Algorithm 2 Data Aggregate

Input: Data packets received from sensor node s_i at CH_i at timestamp (TS_i)
Output: Aggregated Data Packet

1: **for** each DP_i in N **do**
2:    $count \leftarrow 0$;
3:    **if** $p_bit = true$ **then**
4:       Forward to Sink Node
5:    **else**
6:       Apply k-means on DP with $k = CL$
7:       **for** each k_i **do**
8:          **for** each S_j where $j = 1,2,3,...n$ **do**
9:             Calculate variance, $Var_i = \dfrac{(d_i - \mu_i)^2}{l}$ given in 10.4
10:          **end for**
11:       **end for**
12:       Calculate difference in variance of data packets from same source in different clusters given by equation 10.3
13:       **if** $Diff == 1$ **then**
14:          $D \leftarrow$ Aggregate (d_i, d_j)
15:          $count + +$;
16:       **else**
17:          Forward to sink node since packets contain different information
18:       **end if**
19:    **end if**
20: **end for**
21: return count;
22: return D;

10.2 RESULTS AND DISCUSSIONS

The simulation as well as analytical performance analysis along with the network model to support the evaluation of the proposed technique is given in the subsequent sub-sections.

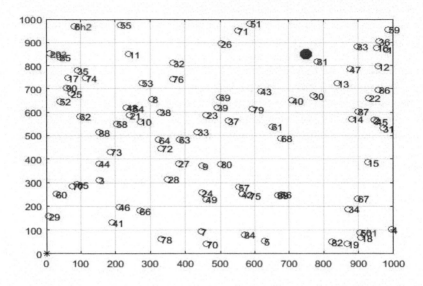

Figure 10.3   Network Model

For performance evaluation of the proposed scheme, an in-door hospital scenario for tier-1 WBAN communication is considered. The hospital building may consist of *n* number of floors with *m* number of patients on each floor with *k* intermediary nodes. As each patient has one sensor node, therefore, the total number of nodes equals number of patients. All the sensor nodes have the same communicational powers and can have P2P multi-hop communication to transmit the data from the source to the sink. Sensor nodes sense and transfer the data to the respective CHs. The data is then transmitted to the nearest fixed node for aggregation. Figure 10.3 shows a network diagram with three CH and an aggregator node. Also, Figure 10.4 depicts how the information flows in the network using the proposed technique.

The proposed protocol for data aggregation is simulated in MATLAB (version 16a). The *n* sensor nodes are divided into clusters. Each CH sends data to the aggregator node. After the process of aggregation, k-means is applied to find the best representative among the data packets from same sensor node. It is then forwarded to the sink node. The proposed technique is assessed using real data set [385]. The data packets with similar variance are aggregated which reduce the number of packets. The experimental results depict higher performance levels of the proposed algorithm when compared to state-of-the-art techniques at different threshold levels. It aids in optimizing energy utilization, total packets aggregated and transmitted, propagation delay and residual energy in compared to OCER [377], EERP [378] and EHDA [376]. The description simulation parameters are listed in Table 10.1.

Discarding redundant data packets from the network yield resource utilization by lowering packet transmissions, energy exhaustion and network congestion.

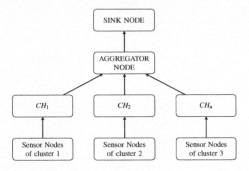

Figure 10.4 Information flow

Table 10.1
Simulation Parameters

Parameters	Values
Minimum threshold value of energy	3J
Packet size	2000 bits
Sensing area	$1000m \times 1000m$
Sink node coordinates (x,y)	(750, 850)
Total sensor nodes (N)	100, 200, 500 and 1000

Figures 10.5 and 10.6 indicate total percentage of data aggregated and total number of packets aggregated, respectively, at different threshold levels. For more threshold value, more change in data packets from the same sensor can be accommodated; therefore, more number of packets can be aggregated.

Next, due to more aggregation in the proposed algorithm with increased threshold values, there is lesser traffic on the network which in turn requires less work done by data communication protocols. Therefore, sensor nodes can preserve their energy levels. As sensor nodes have more energy, they can be alive for longer period of time, hence the longer network lifetime. Figures 10.7 and 10.8 compare the overall energy consumption for a given threshold level and total number of packets aggregated, respectively.

Next, average delay increases with increasing levels of threshold. As the number of packets to be aggregated increases, the process of aggregation takes more time, and hence average delay increases. Moreover, due to reduced number of transmissions average delay reduces due to lower network congestion. Figures 10.9 and 10.10 compare the protocols in terms of average delay (in msec) while aggregating

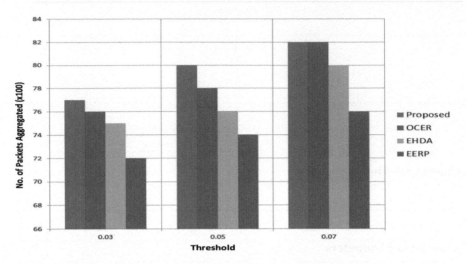

Figure 10.5 Data aggregation (in %) with threshold levels

data at different threshold levels and aggregating increasing number of packets, respectively.

Next, due to reduced network traffic, resource utilization of the network increases. Therefore, the packet delivery ratio improves as the number of transmissions reduces. Figures 10.11 and 10.12 evaluate packet delivery ratio with various threshold levels and total aggregated packets, respectively.

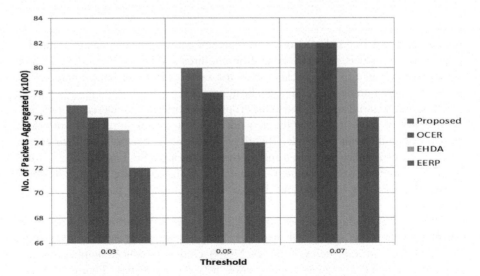

Figure 10.6 No. of packets aggregated with threshold levels

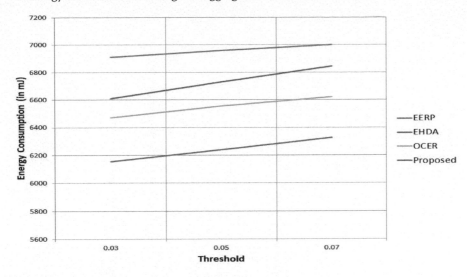

Figure 10.7 Energy consumption with threshold levels

Next, network lifetime is measured by the total number of rounds for which the algorithm runs on the network till the last active node in the network. It is directly proportional to the energy consumption of the sensor network. As the threshold increases, network lifetime decreases due to more packet aggregation in the network and lesser packet re-transmissions. Figures 10.13 and 10.14 evaluate the network lifetime with threshold levels and packet aggregations, respectively.

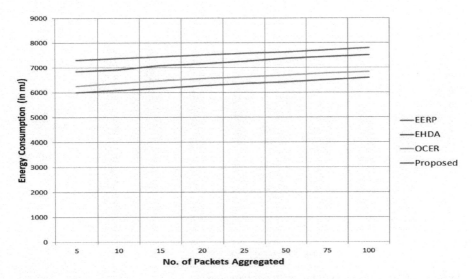

Figure 10.8 Energy consumption with packets aggregated

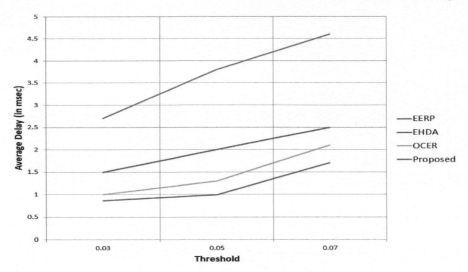

Figure 10.9   Average delay with threshold levels

10.2.1   ANALYTICAL RESULTS

The analytical results of the proposed data reduction and data aggregation algorithms with respect to performance parameters such as data aggregation, energy usage, average propagation delay and network lifetime are discussed below.

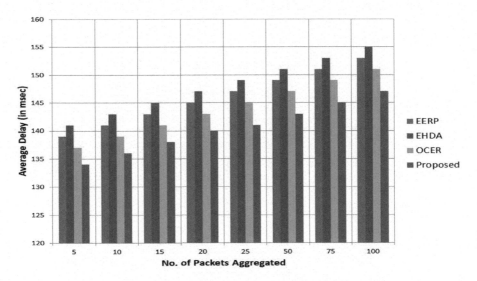

Figure 10.10   Average delay with packets aggregated

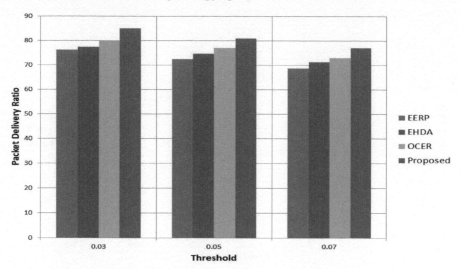

Figure 10.11 Packet delivery ratio with threshold levels

Lemma 1 *Efficient data aggregation depends on temporal correlation and variance between data to reduce redundancy.*

Proof 1 *The proposed protocol considers data for aggregation from same sensor node because reducing the number of redundant data packets before transmitting it to the sink node is necessary for saving resources of the network from exploitation. The data received from the same sensor node is eligible for aggregation as shown*

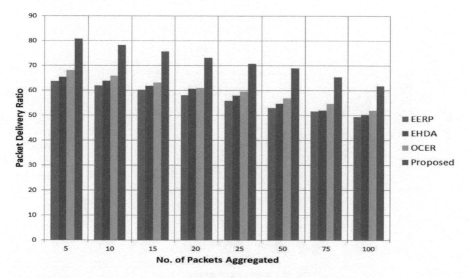

Figure 10.12 Packet delivery ratio with packets aggregated

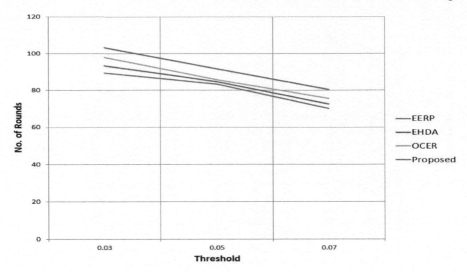

Figure 10.13   Network lifetime with threshold levels

in Equation 10.5. If the variance in data received at different timestamps is below a particular threshold, then the data is similar and should be aggregated.

$$Data_a gg = \begin{cases} 1, & \text{if received from same sensor node} \\ 0, & \text{otherwise} \end{cases} \qquad (10.5)$$

Lemma 2 *Reduction in number of packet transmission reduces energy consumption as well as delay.*

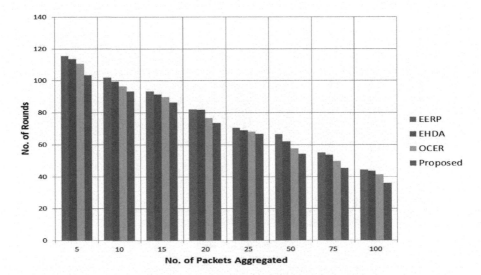

Figure 10.14   Network lifetime with packets aggregated

Proof 2 *As the data are aggregated, lesser number of packets are transmitted which ultimately affect the performance of the aggregator node. Fixed node performs aggregation on the data received from the source nodes. The data from the same sensor node is aggregated depending upon the variance in data. Therefore, lesser number of packets are transmitted from fixed node to sink as compared to sensor node to the fixed node. Therefore, lesser energy is consumed during communication in the network. Further, the total time taken for data transmission is reduced if the data is transmitted via intermediate node which in this case is the aggregator node. This reduces the delay in transmissions and reduces energy usage.*

Lemma 3 *Network lifetime depends on energy usage and packet re-transmissions.*

Proof 3 *Since lesser network energy is consumed, sensor nodes can live for a longer time. Also, the lesser number of re-transmission of messages contributes to optimized packet delivery ratio. This increases the efficiency and performance of the network.*

10.3 CONCLUSIONS AND FUTURE SCOPE

In this chapter, the proposed data aggregation technique is profitably implemented for cost-effective data transmission and energy consumption in WBANs. It uses divide and conquer, k-means and the concept of priority data for aggregating data at the intermediary node. The proposed technique has considered in-door hospital scenario with n sensor nodes on m floors with k intermediary nodes. The respective CH receive data from the sensor nodes. Further, the data from various CH are sent to the near by fixed node. The fixed node performs aggregation by first dividing the data packet into a single unit and then combining the data packets. Then the aggregated data is transmitted from the fixed node to the sink node. Also, the proposed technique transmits the critical data on a priority basis. In order to validate the proposed scheme, experiments have been performed using MATLAB simulator. The experimental results depict the successful implementation of the proposed scheme as it could attain 30% of reduction in total number of packets to be transmitted and consumes up to 63% lesser energy than other techniques, thus helps in improving the overall performance and adoption of WBANs. For future work, a cost-effective route can be found between all intermediary nodes to transmit data to the sink node. Also, the selection of intermediary nodes could be considered for cost-effective data aggregation and data fusion.

11 Case Studies on Implementation of Smart Healthcare across Global Smart Cities

Jagadeesha R Bhat, Omar alfandi, Ahed Abugabah and Jang-Ping Sheu

CONTENTS

DOI: 10.1201/9781003239895-11

11.1 INTRODUCTION

Globally, when the cities are redesigned as smart cities, the smart healthcare and well-being of its citizens will be one of the binding necessities. Smart healthcare is one of the wicked problems of the smart city. In a smart city, there are several challenges with regard to smart healthcare such as ageing population and frequent hospitalizations, increased hospital management cost, patient dissatisfaction, risks involved during patient care and safety of lives during pandemics, etc., which have led to envisaging smart healthcare [386]. Further, the World Health Organization (WHO) has anticipated that there will be a shortage of 18 million healthcare professionals in low- and middle-income countries by 2030 [387]. The only way to address this scarcity and thereby increase the efficiency of patient care is by efficient utilization of available medical facilities. In this regard, smart healthcare would act as a remedy to address the challenges of conventional patient care. One of the benefits of smart healthcare is that it could be extended beyond the walls of the hospital (ex: online consultations) in a cost-effective and resource-efficient way. Besides, the advantages include easier hospital management, better diagnosis, safer and timely care delivery. Considering the above benefits, several global smart cities have begun to upgrade hospitals as smart hospitals with the aim of systematic orchestration of available infrastructure to offer better, uninterrupted healthcare services to their citizens [388].

In recent times, COVID-19 has been contemplated as the greatest contemporary tragedy witnessed all over the globe. Due to COVID-19, the world has lost nearly 4 million people, and 190 million people have got infected [386]. Further, the global economy, healthcare, manufacturing and supply chain process have worst affected due to the outbreak of the pandemic. Every country has deployed all its resources to find a solution to contain the spread of the virus. Yet, an efficient solution to check the transmission is far from reach. However, the world is hopeful about anti-viral vaccine for coronavirus against its various mutations.

In any city, the journey towards smart healthcare begins with the digitalization of health records, smart sensor-based patient monitoring and tracking medical facilities, automation of patient rooms, patient data analysis, intelligent decisions, high-speed wireless networks for data access and an efficient data storage system, etc. In addition, the recent developments in the Internet of Things (IoT), 3D printing, robotic surgery, artificial intelligence (AI), augmented reality (AR), virtual reality (VR), machine learning (ML), deep learning (DL), blockchain, Big data, smart materials, 5G broadband and telemedicine have begun a new paradigm in smart hospitals. These technologies address the long-term goals such as precision and preventive healthcare, overall satisfaction of healthcare stakeholders, optimized functional efficiency and cost reduction [389]. Further, these technologies were extensively useful in the fight against COVID-19. The role of technology in healthcare will ensure that the treatment process shall become deterministic, personalized, efficient in terms of results and well managed. With these objectives, cities have adopted smart healthcare. Further, these technologies were extensively useful in the fight against COVID-19.

However, smart healthcare is subject to several challenges due to the inherent constraints associated with different technologies, patient care procedures, etc. By anticipating the challenges and the scope of ICT in smart healthcare implementation, a few cities around the world have developed the smart hospitals, care models that deserve to be cited.

11.2 SMART HEALTHCARE ASSISTIVE TECHNOLOGIES

Smart healthcare, a.k.a. digital healthcare, is primarily enabled by the smart and green buildings, Information and Communication Technology (ICT), open data, storage, analytics, and automation of the smart city. In this regard, the smart city governments invest diligently in different enablers. For instance, in the year 2020, the USA, the United Kingdom, Japan and Singapore have invested $1B each in their smart city projects. Besides, a survey predicts that global smart healthcare value would increase to USD 128 billion by 2027 [386].

Now, lets us take a brief look at the evolution of smart healthcare [390]. Initially, when the healthcare data was stored in the electronic form for better storage and collection, it was denoted as e-healthcare. In the later phase, when body-worn sensors gathered data and were monitored through mobile devices, m-healthcare evolved. Recently, due to the upgradation of ICT infrastructure of the cities, s-healthcare (smart healthcare) emerged. Anyway, due to the inception of technology

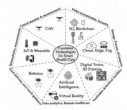

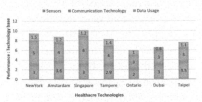

(a) Candidate Technologies for Smart Healthcare

(b) Technology Vs. Performance

Figure 11.1   A brief look at the enablers of smart healthcare technology with regard to a smart city. (a) Candidate technologies for smart healthcare (b) Technology vs. Performance

in healthcare, patient care will change from disease specific to patient-specific. To be specific, instead of providing episode-based treatment, offer continuous health monitor for overall health management.

Consequently, the dealing with the patient data should orient towards personalized management than general management. Recently, during the ongoing pandemic, the smart technologies have contributed enormously to the quick detection and decision-making in smart healthcare. Refer to Fig. 11.1(a) for a brief look at the enablers of smart healthcare technology with regard to a smart city [391, 392]. Similarly, in Fig. 11.1(b), we have compared the broad technologies for healthcare in different smart cities by adopting the data in [393].

11.2.1   INTERNET OF THINGS (IOTS)

IoT is an efficient digital healthcare component due to its simplicity of device architecture, versatility and low cost. Earlier, RFIDs assisted in detecting human movements during hospitalization, homecare, etc., however, in a limited geographical area [394]. IoTs for healthcare consist of wearable devices such as smartwatches, or sensor-based wraps to monitor glucose level, heartbeat, sleep pattern, muscle activities, etc., which are termed as Medical Internet of Things (MIoT) [395]. Generally, data from these sensors will be sent to the cloud (internet) or directly to the monitoring unit (through short-range communication systems). The data transmission will be through one or multiple wireless technologies, namely, Bluetooth, Wi-Fi, LoRa, LTE and 5G.

The IoT and wearable devices facilitated remote monitoring of COVID-19 patients by wirelessly transmitting the temperature, heartbeat, oxygen level, physical movements, sleep pattern, location, etc., continuously to the monitoring station through the internet and reduced the burden on healthcare facilities. In addition, smart sensors and IoT devices are of immense use during maintaining the social distances to alert people when they are too nearby, which also assists indirectly in contact tracking and enforcing stay home quarantine rules. Moreover, remote healthcare and telemedicine would not have been so successful without these wearable devices. However, due to the limited storage, power and processing capabilities, IoT devices work in amalgamation with the cloud computing system and Apps for further data processing, analysis and storage.

11.2.2 ARTIFICIAL INTELLIGENCE (AI)

AI is the driving force behind the healthcare devices that behave smart to assist doctors in clinical diagnosis. The AI, along with the ML/DL and reinforcement learning, enables early detection of cancer from pathology or radiology images, stroke detection by analysing the brain signals, online chatbots to assist patients in receiving online recommendations and many more [393]. In general, AI assists in data analysis, classification, prediction, decision-making and providing recommendations in smart healthcare.

AI is the prime technology that has been well exploited during this pandemic. AI has been used for massive and quick response in detecting the infection, analysing the rate of spread, and decision requirements. Therefore, AI and its sub-fields, namely, ML, DL, neural networks have been used worldwide, especially in the analysis of chest and lung images, understand the minute possibilities of corona infection in patients with or without significant symptoms [57]. For instance, face and mask detection, DL-based dashboards to predict the casualties, etc. Nevertheless, the biggest challenge with regard to the AI systems was the availability of data to train the agents to predict the future. Since the accuracy of prediction depends on how well the system is trained, only a few major cities could develop the efficient AI-based management systems.

11.2.3 BIG DATA ANALYTICS

All patient data that arrive through wearable devices, smart homes, need to be classified, sorted, processed for storage and analysis either at the edge, fog or cloud storage as the massive data will have varying formats. Several countries have maintained electronic health records (EHR) for efficient management of patient data. However, to enforce the security of big data, a distributed blockchain mechanism is much recommended.

As seen in the previous section, the IoT and wearable patches send vast and vivid data types, thus posing a significant challenge at the cloud for process and analysis. Especially, due to the surge in the number of positive Corona cases all over the world, cloud and edge computing experienced a massive influx of data than ever before in recent times. Thus, to manage this big data, several cloud management firms deployed AI and DL to analyse and classify the data and to make quick decisions during the process and storage. The big data from several medical IoT devices were initially processed at the device itself and later sent to the edge platforms to avoid the huge delay involved in cloud computing.

Robotics: Many smart hospitals use robots to educate future surgeons, guide patients regarding their disease, track hospital facilities and for surgeries. In the case of robotic surgery, the surgeons control the robotic arms, which could reach hard to operate areas of the body with precision and ease. Nevertheless, patient safety and regulations are concerns. During the pandemic, robots have been used to serve medicine, provide a suggestion and monitor patients in hospitals to avoid direct human contact.

11.2.4   UNMANNED AERIAL VEHICLES (UAV)

UAV assists in the logistics of medical facilities like first aid boxes, vital organs for transplant to distant areas within a few minutes. In order to avoid direct human-to-human contact, robots were used during the pandemic. Further, the robots were used to deliver food, assist visitors in the hospital, caregiving the quarantined patients and supply goods. In addition, UAVs were extensively used for crowd monitoring and aerial temperature measurements. The digital twins have functioned as data loggers in the cloud and are used to train the medical teams remotely and transfer certain skills digitally.

11.2.5   5G AND BEYOND 5G (B5G)

The three key features of 5G, which include enhanced mobile broadband (eMBB), ultra-Reliable Low Latency Communication (uRLLC) and massive Machine Type Communication (mMTC), support smart healthcare in several ways. For instance, the success of robotic surgery depends on extremely low latency (1ms or lower) and the transfer of massive data requiring a very high data rate (Gbps). Further, when there exists a high density of wearable devices, networking them requires massive bandwidth (order of GHz). Since 5G shall support these requirements to a certain extent, it becomes a potential candidate. The different smart healthcare components such as robotic surgery, connected wearable devices, telemedicine that requires varying quality of service shall be accommodated in one network by performing network slicing. Figure 11.2 shows a proposed scenario of network slices, where each virtual network slice will offer different network features such as ultra-low latency, high

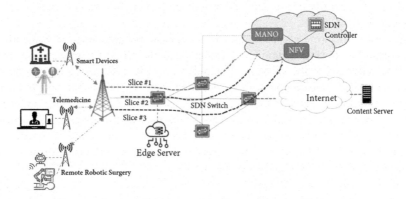

Figure 11.2   A scenario of 5G network slicing for smart healthcare

density and high data rate. Nevertheless, holographic video transfer in the case of remote healthcare, latency for certain events having min and max requirements will demand B5G or 6G networks.

11.3 SMART HEALTHCARE IN GLOBAL SMART CITIES

In this section, we highlight the key smart healthcare practices implemented by different global smart cities as a case study.

Let's see in general, how the smart cities have explored their smart infra in making the lives of people better in selected cities globally.

11.3.1 ONTARIO, CANADA

The first city we consider is Ontario (province) smart city, Canada. The city of Ontario has invested its resources in building Canada's first smart hospital. At the Vaughan region, Mackenzie Vaughan Hospital (MVH) is a state-of-the-art smart hospital that has integrated internet and ICT solutions to deliver better patient care [396].

At MaKenzie smart hospital, IoT plays a key role in patient treatment, communication between patients and caregivers (i.e. doctor, nurse) and management of wards. It exploits web technologies in extending healthcare facilities to remote patients and appointment bookings. In addition, the hospital uses the ideology of smart infrastructure in which operation rooms, patient wards have facilities like automated lighting, temperature settings and control of the door.

11.3.1.1 Remote Healthcare

Now, let us consider one of the smart healthcare projects in detail. The MaKenzie hospital uses a collaborative online platform, 'weHealth', to connect its various stakeholders such as patients, doctors, nurses, pharmacy, hospital amenities and citizens through the internet to achieve efficiency in healthcare service through collaborations in a secure way. Further, this platform even educates people to encourage them in self-care. For example, patients can upload their temperature or blood pressure into the system through weHealth mobile app and get suggestions from the database, which is maintained centrally by the hospital. Next, due to the electronic patient data repository called Epic EMR and intra-hospital linkage between different departments, the patients can receive unified audio-visual instructions and personalized telehealth services. Further, MyChart platform enables healthcare providers and patients to access the test reports, upload patient data and schedule follow-up appointments online through a secured login system.

Another initiative of the hospital is called virtual hospital, where all patient consultations are pushed to the online mode, and only the patients in need of emergency care will be directed to the actual hospital. Here, initially, the person in need of healthcare services could connect to the doctors and caregivers online, and only if further treatment is necessary shall visit the hospital. The virtual hospital concept reduces the risk of infections, saves time and reduces the burden on the hospital's infrastructure without compromising the quality of service.

11.3.1.2 COVID-19 Action

Several cities in Canada including Ontario, uses COVID Alert app for contact tracing. The said app uses the Bluetooth signal and exchanges a random code with the nearby phones if the COVID Alert app and Bluetooth are ON in both the mobile phones. Later, the random codes will be used to determine if the user had any close contact with the person who tested positive for Corona virus. When a person is diagnosed with COVID-19, the data will be uploaded to the system that maps the person to his random code. The app will enable other users to determine the status of contact with the help of these random codes exchanged through Bluetooth. Consequently, any person who identifies himself as close contact with an infected person shall remain cautious for the next 15 days. This app will not exclusively store the location of the user, and the data will be erased after 15 days.

11.3.1.3 AI for Prediction

Determining the spread of the novel coronavirus was essential at the earliest when COVID-19 out broke. In this regard, BlueDot, a Toronto's digital healthcare provider company, anticipated the spread of the coronavirus at Wuhan, China. Their prediction involves data from several sources such as population, medical reports, news bulletins, etc., and uses big data analytics and AI on the gathered data to generate the predictions. Drones were used to reduce human contact during the supply of essentials during the pandemic. For instance, GlobalMedic deployed its drones in Beausoleil, Ontario to supply the essentials during the pandemic. Figure 11.3 shows the comparison of various smart technologies used in cities.

Technologies	Potentials	Challenges	Use Cases
IoT & Wearables	Improved care delivery, Low Power Consumption, Ease of networking, Cost efficient	Miniaturization, Radiation, Burns, Diverse connectivity interfaces	Remote monitoring, Medical device integration, Self- evaluation,
UAV	Reachable to challenging areas	Cost, Durability, Safety	Emergency delivery of medical care
Beyond 5G	High data rate, Low latency	Bandwidth and Coverage for advanced Virtual surgery	Support for massive medical IoT devices, Health App,
Cloud, Edge, Fog	Economical, Scalable, Large Database for EHR	Latency, Security	Storage of EHR, Edge/ Fog system at patient side data processing
Smart Structures, 3D Printing	Energy efficiency, Improved Communications, Pre surgical modelling,	Cost, Compatibility issues of Printed body parts	Efficient patientcare, 3D printed body parts, Pre-surgical analysis
Artificial Intelligence	Improved clinical decisions, Hospital process assistance (patient, nurse, and doctors)	Training Data, Privacy	AI for image analysis, Critical patient alarming
Robotics, Digital Twins	Surgical assistance, Patientcare, Treatment simulation	Patient Safety, Regulations	Robotic Surgery, Patient guidance, and Monitoring
Telemedicine	Reduced hospital visit, Low risk of infections	Network connectivity.	Online medical consultation, Routine check-ups

Figure 11.3   Eco-system of smart healthcare: potentials and challenges

11.3.2 NEW YORK CITY, USA

As a part of its smart city program, New York has promoted several digital healthcare service providers to facilitate an easy transition towards an electronic and cloud-based smart healthcare system. We review two hospitals in New York City that have integrated digital technologies into their patient care.

11.3.2.1 E-Awareness

Mount Sinai hospital provides customized and disease-specific guidance to each in-patient through a customized software using a bedside tablet PC. The patients can access certain specific content and video conference features to learn more based on their disease profile. Further, remote patient care is assisted through a translation app and handwriting analysis that removes language barriers between patient and care provider. These digital facilities have saved the nurse's time and reduced the re-admissions due to better comfort and faster healing [397].

11.3.2.2 COVID-19 Action

The United States of America is one of the worst-hit nations on earth due to COVID-19. Therefore, we discuss the smart healthcare measure taken by other cities of the USA as well. In a recent development, due to the outbreak of COVID-19, the hospital uses Google Nest Smart home cameras inside patient rooms to provide bi-directional virtual communication. With the help of remote monitoring and instructions, the nurses can avoid redundant contact with the patients to curtail the spread of the infection. Secondly, New York-Presbyterian Hospital, in association with Philips, has introduced a remote health monitoring scheme, where doctors provide telehealthcare to the patients through Philips eCareCoordinator. The eCareCompanion platform runs in a tablet PC, interfaced with several medical instruments and wearable devices to capture patients' health status such as blood pressure, temperature, etc., and remotely update the doctor. Later, doctors provide online suggestions based on patient data and subjective interactions. This online platform-based service model will provide cost-effective patient care without the need to visit the hospital. ML and robotics have been used to achieve efficiency in hospital administration tasks such as patient ID assignment, billing and insurance processing in collaboration with Work-Fusion, a robotics solution provider. For instance, to ensure the correct coding of patients and avoid incorrect mapping of medical reports, robots with natural language processing capabilities have been trained with ML algorithms that can read and analyse key data from charts to avoid any mismatching. These robots can also read the data from invoices of different formats, which reduces the burden on the administrative staff.

11.3.2.3 COVID Visualizers

The John Hopkin hospital developed a real-time dashboard that gives regular updates about the number of recovered, infected and fatalities globally from various sources [398]. It acts as the main source of real-time information, globally. Further, Microsoft has developed Bingmap, which summarizes Corona cases by aggregating the data from WHO and CDC in the USA. Similarly, in the UK, a public COVID visualizer gives the statistics of active, recovered and deaths in a chosen region of the United Kingdom [399]. Further, Google has developed its dashboard to provide information regarding pandemics [400]. Coronavirus checker, an internet application that allows people to analyse their symptoms and understand the level of risk, was developed by Emory University school of medicine, Georgia [401]. The virtual reality tools were used to visualize the impact of coronavirus on human organs. For example, George Washington University Hospital developed a model of lungs using virtual reality to study the impact of the virus and the damage it causes to the inner walls of the lungs. New York University developed an AI tool to predict which mildly infected patients will worsen the infection based on their symptoms and body conditions. The tool used predictive analytics to train the AI system that used data samples of 53 COVID-19 patients and gave recommendations about the patients who will become too sick [402]. In certain cities in the USA, online food delivery shops used robots to deliver food to the customers to avoid human contact during the crisis.

AI was used to analyse the chest X-ray and study the amount of lung damage which determines the possibility of risk of coronavirus. This system was developed by Princeton University. The X-ray images were accurately predicted by the AI system about the chances of getting the infection as accurate as the findings of a CT image [403]. Remote monitoring the patients has been assisted by a wireless device Emerald, an invention of MIT researchers. This wireless device transmits wireless signals that efficiently collect vital parameters such as no. of breaths, movement of chest walls and sleep patterns to report to the AI system in the wireless device. The AI agent will analyse these received signals to assist the remote doctors in better decision-making about the treatment procedures. It even assists in the early detection of insomnia and several other respiratory disorders. In Chicago, the Northwestern Memorial hospital has deployed stamp-sized medical wearable sensors to record the body temperature and oxygen level for the early detection of COVID-19. The sensor technology has been developed by the joint efforts of Northwestern University and a group of other scientists. To avoid direct contact between healthcare professionals and patients, Massachusetts General Hospital uses intelligent robots to serve COVID positive patients at their ward, including temperature monitor, oxygen level, delivery of food and medicine.

11.3.3 TAMPERE CITY, FINLAND

Tampere, one of the six smart cities of Finland, has taken extensive measures to excel in smart healthcare by associating with research institutes, healthcare providers, fitness equipment manufacturers and start-ups to deliver digital healthcare services to all its citizens by 2025. Tampere University hospital is a major player in well-being and smart healthcare facilities in Tampere smart city. Let's consider some of the initiatives here. Tays RDI centre and Philips offer AI-enabled smart cardiac imaging solutions to assist doctors in better decision-making. It also provides OmaTays, a mobile app through which diabetes patients can upload their daily sugar level, and other vital health parameters online from their phone or tablet PC. The patient data integrates automatically with a medical database named-ENDO maintained by the hospital. By that, the doctors can provide timely online feedback to the patients which saves time and resources [404].

11.3.3.1 Online Interpreter

Tampere has several experts who do not speak Finnish, making it difficult for the nurses to understand patients' sufferings. To assist such patients and hospital staff with a language disability, Tampere translation app named Tulka provides online translation services with the help of an interpreter who will translate the patient's audio to Finnish online.

11.3.3.2 Remote Health Counselling by Chat

A healthcare chat box allows students at the upper secondary schools to discuss their health issues remotely through the online chat system and gets solutions. Further, as a part of this digital health service, Tampere has developed a database 'Omaolo' that realizes the minute and specific conditions of a patient and provides patient-specific recommendations, prescriptions or notifies emergency care online. This feature has made patients get customized solutions at one place rather than searching for pieces of general solutions scattered all over the internet.

11.3.3.3 COVID-19 Action

Telia company assisted the Tampere city govt., in detecting the mobility pattern of citizens anonymously to curb the spread of COVID-19. The Telia crowd used mobile network data anonymously to track the groups and individuals. By this, the government can take precautionary measures to control the groups to prevent the spread of the pandemic.

11.3.4 TAIPEI CITY, TAIWAN

Taiwan being a small island nation offers one of the best healthcare facilities in the world. With regard to smart healthcare, it has several schemes such as telemedicine, remote patient care, robotics for patient awareness, AR-based entertainment for people with limited mobility, etc., to name a few. The department of social welfare in association with Origin Wireless Inc. has introduced ML-based elderly activity detection for smart homes and hospitals. The proposed technology does not require any wearable devices, instead uses Wi-Fi signals to detect the change in the radiation pattern of electromagnetic signals generated by a Wi-Fi antenna when the person being monitored moves or breaths inside the room. The cloud-based ML algorithms analyse these movements by comparing the radiation pattern of the room under different mobility conditions, and remotely alerts the caretaker or the nurse for the necessary action [405].

11.3.4.1 Telemedicine

Taipei City Hospital serves the patients in the remote area of Lienjiang County through telemedicine consultations and provides home care by using the ICT infrastructure of the smart city. Especially, the tele-recommendation project targets patients with cataract surgery. During the guided remote surgery, the doctors from Taipei City Hospital supervise the surgery through video conferences while the surgery is conducted by the Lienjiang County healthcare professionals at their medical facility. Similarly, patients with dementia also receive remote recommendations as a part of this collaborative project [406].

11.3.4.2 Robotics in Healthcare

Taipei City Hospital uses an AI-based smart multi-function robot that can perform face detection to assist people in eye testing and service satisfaction survey. A robot with feature extraction capability scans the eyes of the patient in real time and collects the eye data. The collected data is processed and analysed by AI algorithms as part of the eye test and suggests accurate vision corrections. This robotic eye test reduces the doctors' load [405]. Apart from these, the city government and Vicon Healthcare international have jointly introduced self-operated automatic nervous monitoring and self-health management system at the community sports centre. In this, a smart ECG machine captures an athlete's cardiac signal and analyses it with computer technology to detect hidden illnesses like chest tightness, breathlessness and poor blood circulation. This technology can reduce the chances of injuries such as potential cardiac arrest during sports activities.

11.3.4.3 COVID-19 Action

Furthermore, Taiwan used big data from EHR, and the immigration department to map citizens' health and travel history to detect the potential COVID-19 patients. For a quick detection of the positive cases, AI was used to analyse the pulmonary X-ray. In addition, IoT and AI-based Microsoft systems detect the presence of face masks and body temperature automatically during the screening test. During the onset of the pandemic, Taiwan initiated emergency measures at the earliest to stop the spread of infection. It used IoT, AI, to routinely screen the individuals to reduce the burden on frontline staff. For instance, Yonghe Cardinal Tien Hospital installed Microsoft's multi-sensory monitoring device to automatically determine the temperature and the presence of face mask of every individual using AI during the daily screening procedure. The facial images from the AI system and sensor data are processed and analysed in a local IoT edge device. This feature enables mapping temperature to the person by recognizing his image in the presence of a facial mask. Next, Taiwan used Big data, generated from its EHR and immigration data to map citizens with health conditions and their travel history. This enabled the COVID task force to track people with potential risks. AI algorithms drastically reduce the test time and improve the accuracy and thereby enables quick decisions that can reduce the harm. As a start-up company, iWEECARE introduced the smart thermometer patch to be worn on the body.

11.3.5 AMSTERDAM CITY, NETHERLANDS

The city of Amsterdam has incorporated remote healthcare through IoT, AI for monitoring surgery, ML for efficient risk detection of patients in its healthcare projects with the support of existing as well as start-up companies to emerge as a leader in smart healthcare in Europe [407]. In order to improve the health and living conditions of the people of Amsterdam, the Amsterdam Health & Technology Institute (AHTI) was setup to initiate smart city projects. One of the projects (ATHENA) which provides remote healthcare with the help of a smart wrist-band. It enables a patient with hypertension to self-monitor their blood pressure and connect to a mobile app. This system provides personalized treatment and medications to the patient with the aid of a mobile triage. Further, a medical practitioner can access the patient data over the internet to cross-examine the reliability of the mobile App's suggestions.

11.3.5.1 AI-Assisted Surgery

Amsterdam UMC, a leading healthcare provider in Netherlands uses AI to monitor surgeries. An AI-based 'black box' acts as an observer in the operation room during the surgery and alerts the surgeons in case of anomalies that could not be detected easily otherwise. The black box even assists doctors in the post-surgery analysis. The AI system in the black box has been trained with instances of surgery that assist in providing recommendations or while raising an alert. Further, Amsterdam UMC also uses the black box in surgical education to train potential surgeons by providing a detailed analysis of each case. The SAS Platform, a healthcare technology provider, facilitates the integration of computer vision, predictive analysis and AI by that the doctors can make accurate decisions regarding the tumours of cancer patients, which otherwise requires high expertise in analysing the CT images manually. Similarly, Pacmed is another organization that works with Amsterdam UMC to provide AI and ML-based solutions to analyse urinary tract infections, diabetes, hypertension, etc., by collecting patient data during their visit to the doctor.

'Hospital of the Future' is a key project between Philips and Dutch Rijnstate Hospital, Netherlands to implement ICT infrastructure in healthcare services. Especially, the doctors can provide service from a remote virtual command room with the aid of Philips technology IntelliVue Guardian Solution. This remote monitoring system collects vital data from remote patients and transmits the data over the internet to the command room (Rijnstate) for continuous monitoring. Further, it facilitates in-hospital patient monitoring.

11.3.5.2 COVID-19 Action

In recent developments, during the outbreak of COVID-19, Philips along with the Netherlands Ministry of Health and a network of hospitals have developed an on-line portal to securely share COVID-19 patient's radiology, pathology reports, which facilitates the distribution of patient load among different hospitals in the country. Further, Aura Aware, a start-up company, has developed a smart social distancing device based on the Lidar sensor to alert people to maintain social distance. It uses laser technology to measure the distance and alerts through audio-visual notifications. Altogether, the use of AI, IoT, Computer vision and data sciences has made Amsterdam a leading smart health city.

11.3.6 DUBAI, UAE

Smart City projects in Dubai have seen tremendous progress in all aspects including mobility, infrastructure and healthcare. Mobile communication, digital tools and the rise of ICT have made mHealth and eHealth a very affordable and convenient healthcare services in Dubai. All hospitals in Dubai collect patients' data in electronic form which can be accessed by any hospital in Dubai and run predictive analytics for advanced risk detection [408].

11.3.6.1 Robotics in Healthcare

In Latifa Hospital, patients will receive their medication from the robot. The robot will read the barcode on the prescription and dispense the appropriate medicine to the patient at a rate of nine medicines within a minute. The robot can process 35,000 different medicines. This automation can greatly reduce the risk of erroneous drug delivery. American Hospital in Dubai has implemented Robotics Surgery to treat patients with severe complications which offers a reduced risk of infections, precise incision and eases the process as a robot's wrist can reach any part of the body along with the support of computer vision. At Sheikh Khalifa Medical City, robot-assisted knee surgeries have gained attention, where the surgeon operates the patient's body with the help of fine instruments held by a robotic arm. A camera fitted to the instruments provides a 360-degree view which facilitates the doctor to guide the surgical instruments of the robotic arm with precision. In addition, Universal Hospital treats children with the social disorder (Autism) with small-sized robots. With the help of artificial intelligence algorithms, these robots can be trained to learn a child's mood and respond accordingly.

11.3.6.2 AI for Health Prediction

Smart Dubai's AI Lab in association with IBM, Dubai hospital, and three other hospitals have implemented AI-based high precision nurses (AI systems) that diagnose the patients based on the pre-fed vital parameters such as temperature, pulse, etc., and predicts the patient's future health and suggests precautions. A major feature of this AI nurse consists of monitoring the health condition of the patients in the intensive care unit and predicts the possibility of patient's recovery. Amazingly, these predictions can be done as early as 20 hours before the actual event with more than 90% accuracy. This enables doctors to implement swift actions to save patient's life.

11.3.6.3 3D Printing

The 3D models assist the doctors in planning the surgery well as they could visualize the entire area to be operated on, decide the size of the incision, implants, etc. Dubai

Health Authority innovation centre and Sinterex Inc have joined hands in printing 3D models of the patient organs to assist the doctors in the pre-surgical analysis. In this process, first, an image processing software will segment the MRI images to precisely choose the target area to be operated such as Aortic valves, jaws, skull, etc. Then, the chosen area will be 3D printed and analysed to get a better insight.

11.3.6.4   UAV for Remote Health

UAVs are used to supply first aid medical supplies during an emergency. A person can get such an emergency service by requesting through his smartphone app. Upon receiving the request, the controlling station monitored by a remote caregiver will view the location and condition of the person through a smartphone camera and send the suitable first aid medical supplies through a UAV. At the receiving end, the patient will also get suggestions regarding the procedure of self-first aid through the smartphone from the remote caregiver. Once the treatment is done, the UAV will fly back to the remote centre. Due to these modern healthcare facilities, Dubai stands at the leading position in e-healthcare tourism in the world.

11.3.6.5   COVID-19 Action

A self-operating robot deployed in the public area will detect the symptoms of the coronavirus and communicate the information over the internet. With the help of IoT and AI, the robot can assist in the contactless screening of people.

11.3.6.6   Contact Tracing

UAE used ALHOSN UAE app to determine the close contact of a person with a corona-positive patient using Bluetooth if both are using the similar app. The users' travel history will be saved on the phone which will be accessed by the authority when the user will be at risk or cause potential risk for the rest using the health information uploaded to the app. In addition, this app integrates the information of self-quarantined people, their whereabouts and contact tracing app. Further, a chatbot as a virtual doctor facilitates people to take a survey regarding their own health, possible symptoms and travel history to detect the possibility of risk. In another instance, a taxi dashboard-based AI system was deployed to monitor every passenger in the taxi to determine the proper usage of face masks and physical distance between the co-passengers.

To prevent the possible infection due to healthcare personal, special attention was paid to sanitize the roads. Self-guided robots were used that could analyse the movement and spray the solvent. Similarly, UAVs that could detect human movement were also used to sprinkle the sanitizer on the streets when people move on the street. Further, elevator switches were fitted with infrared sensors that detect the finger at least from a distance of 3cm, thus alleviating the need to touch the buttons to minimize the risk of infection. A sensor-based technology deployed by the Meta Touch, a firm of UAE University's Science and Innovation Park, consists of thermal cameras to detect the individuals and the physical spacing between them to enforce safe distancing.

11.3.6.7 Testing

A laser technology–based non-invasive Diffractive Phase Interferometry (DPI) has been used to test the blood samples at a massive rate to detect the virus much quicker than the swab test.

11.3.7 SINGAPORE CITY, SINGAPORE

Singapore has a rapidly ageing population in the world. To take good care of these populations, there is a shortage of human resources. Therefore, the Singapore government has initiated several smart healthcare projects under the umbrella of the smart country project [409].

11.3.7.1 Smart-Health Assist (SHA)

This project mainly involves providing remote care to patients using the city's smart communication facilities. To be particular, it provides telemedicine that involves the deployment of IoT sensors and wearable devices at the patient side to monitor heart activity, blood pressure and skin glucose patches. Patients with memory issues such as dementia have been provided with sensors having localization features (i.e. GPS) to track their location without violating their privacy norms. Besides, the project also deals with the installation of pill sensors at the patients' end and collects the vital patient body parameters remotely through the internet for analysis. For children with acute heart problems, KK Women's and Children's Hospital use computer simulation and 3D printing technology to build an accurate 3D model of the heart from its 2D scanned images. These help doctors plan the surgery in a better way. Tan Tok Seng smart hospital has several best practices that integrate ICT technologies and healthcare services. It has initiated an official scheme C3 (command, control, and communications) as a major step towards becoming a smart hospital. An online hospital monitoring system maps every patient to the available beds in real time, to get complete information of available hospital resources at any point in time. Further, the efficiency of workflow has been improved by an IoT system that receives data from various functional units of the hospital where centralized monitor and control are executed. Woodland smart hospital has integrated AI, IoT and Robotics to provide the highest level of patient care in the country. The IoT system collects data from wristbands, bedside units of the patient inside the hospital from remote locations. The AI system will investigate the data and assist the doctors in better decision-making. Further, Robots will assist in the delivery of foods to patients, sterilization of medical equipment and automation of a few other sectors of the hospital.

11.3.7.2 Smart Rehabilitation

It is done through robotics and VR programs. For instance, the Lokomat rehabilitation device learns about the patient's gait pattern and provides a real-time walking experience through VR, thereby assists in better rehabilitation.

11.3.7.3 COVID-19 Action

The government of Singapore took technology aid such as automated thermal scanners, self-access chatbots and mobile app for contact tracing, etc., in combating COVID-19. One such mobile app is TraceTogether that uses Bluetooth to communicate with similar nearby devices and stores the contact information locally in an encrypted form. Later, if the user tests positive for the coronavirus, then his phone can be used (with authorization) to track his historical close contacts during the past 21 days. In the fight against COVID-19, the smart nation project of Singapore has the following five main objectives, namely, AI and robots for COVID-19 frontline workers, AI for contact tracing, robots for surveillance, data analysis for better tourism and smart sensors for resource consumption.

11.3.7.4 TraceTogether Contact Tracing App

The mobile-based app uses Bluetooth to exchange an anonymized secret code among similar mobile devices installed with TraceTogether app when both the mobiles are in close proximity of Bluetooth coverage. These secret codes will be saved securely in each of these devices. In case, any of the users get infected in the future, by unlocking the secret code (with consent), all the mobile users who were in close proximity shall be alerted about the possibility of being infected. In this system, the data will be stored for a duration of 25 days, and later it will be deleted by default. This contact tracing app really helped Singapore in the early detection and containment of the infection.

11.4 GLOBAL ANECDOTES OF COVID-19

a) **India**: Recently, India witnessed the largest number of cases reported globally during the second wave, despite the stringent actions taken in the form of national lockdown for nearly 50 days during the first wave. When the country began to implement actions to monitor people in public places, a start-up firm Staqu has developed an AI-based thermal scanning camera that can identify people within a region of 100 meters. The camera alerts the monitoring system through its AI-powered JARVIS analyser when it detects the body temperature of any person greater than 37 degree Celsius. On the other hand, companies such as Tata Consultancy Services, Qure.ai in Mumbai city have integrated AI algorithms to chest X-rays (as similarly done in many other global cities) to identify the opacities in the lung which is the main indicator of the infection. Further, the AI algorithm of Qure.ai can also find the extent of infection in already infected patients which assists in determining the course of treatment and deciding the contact traces.

For instance, if the person has got infected 3 days earlier, but has developed the symptoms just a day before, then all his contacts from the past 3 days should be identified at least [410]. The administration of smart cities of Hyderabad, Cyberabad, and Rachakonda and Telangana have adopted AI in the CCTV cameras to identify the people who do not wear the mask in public places. This automated system sends alert messages to the police to initiate the penalty.

Since, finding a new medicine is time-consuming, analysing the existing drugs and altering their purpose such that to inhibit the action of the coronavirus is the main target of the pharmaceutical industry. In this regard, AI has been used in drug analysis to improve the efficiency of medicine by redefining the objectives of medicine and its molecules using AI for a speedy recovery as done by IIT Delhi. In another instance, Tata Consultancy Services, a major information technology provider for the healthcare sector and Prayas health group, have developed a prediction model to determine the growth of viruses in urban settings. The model used digital twins which fundamentally apply AI algorithms to using real-time data such as average contact durations, number of contacts a person had, risk factors, age, gender, average population, etc., to predict the evolution of the infection [411].

Kerala is another state which was the epic centre of coronavirus in South India. To mitigate the spread of infection by safeguarding the frontline workers, Asimov Robotics deployed its humanoids to dispense the hand sanitizers, deliver medicines to the patients in the isolation wards in its hospitals and to clean the patient rooms. Further, the team of Indian Institute of technology and Stanford University Alumni have deployed a robot named Robo Sapien to ionize the coronavirus and thereby disinfect the public spaces and facilities. Robo-Doc is another robot deployed in hospitals that moves into the COVID wards to measure the temperature and facilitates virtual visits by the doctors from remote rooms. Another example of the usage of robots for patient care is 'Mitra', a doctor-friendly robot developed by *Invento* robotics company in Bangalore. The Mitra robots in Yathara hospital, Noida and Fortis Hospital, Bangalore assists the doctors in measuring patient's vital parameters, takes their photo, contact details for future reference, interacting with patients through its facial recognition and AI capabilities, do the screening of people who enter the hospital, connects patients to their families from the intensive care unit to make the patients emotionally connected. The same firm installed C-Astra robots in Apollo hospital, Bangalore to screen those patients and to sanitize the rooms using UV-C lamps while moving around. Further, Indiana hospital has used cleaning bots to clean the patient rooms. Moreover, tall robots (90cm) height were used in AIIMS hospital, Delhi for similar purposes. Aarogyasetu, 'GoCoronaGo' and 'Sampark-o-meter' have also been developed for contact tracing by the Indian Institute of Science (IISc), Bangalore and IITs.

b) **South Korea**: To detect the presence of active patients, a government app named Corona 100 m will collect peoples' location information through their Smartphone sensor location. Then, the location of infected patients (not the identity) will be published online and mobile-based alert messages are sent to other people in the surrounding to avoid the possibility of contact. The Corona 100 m app will alert the people who are within the 100-m distance of the COVID-19-positive patients.

The users' mobility was traced with the help of three references, namely, mobile network providers, credit card usage location and usage of transportation card in public locations. This platform uses data from the smart city project in association with MOLIT a govt., organization. A confirmed patient's travel history will be revealed by the mobile operator including the location of the credit card usage. This open data to the COVID-19 investigating agency helped to track the potential risk patients and to isolate them. These apps use big data analysis extensively to extract the location data of a crowd.

c) **Israel**: The government of Israel used a citizen's mobile location to track an infected person and to trace his close contacts. This information is sent to the mobile phone of the people as a text message who should observe self-quarantine.

Further, Maccabi healthcare service, Israel used AI on the medical records collected from the hospitals during the earlier visit of the patients. The AI system assists to classify the patients into different risk groups of coronavirus infection by analysing their pre-medical histories. Based on this analysis, the high-risk population is alerted to take extreme care to avoid the contract of the virus. In addition, Israel aerospace industries developed an AI model to monitor the condition of COVID-19 patients using ML and big data. The predictions generated by the AI system is then communicated to the medical staff for suitable action. In addition, Israel introduced the smart commuting app 'Moovit' to mobilize its population during the crisis. The cloud-based app offers mobility as a service (MaaS) where it provides customized transport facilities to commuters based on their selection of mode of transport. The app uses intelligent routing algorithms to determine the efficient route from the source to the destination while avoiding infected areas.

Tel Aviv used heatmap visualization to identify the locations having high risk due to the asymptomatic population using AI. The heatmap updates automatically in real time based on the movement of the people to alert the city authorities about the concentration of the asymptomatic population. The Spark Beyond system integrates all buildings, where data from a transport hub, Open Street maps and from several other points is integrated and analysed by the AI system to generate the heatmap. This assists in implementing suitable restrictive measures on peoples' movement.

d) **Germany**: Initially, Germany used a centralized database where all data was reported from the people to determine the possible contact cases. However, using a centralized database lacked privacy which made the authorities discontinue it. The recent mobile-based Corona Warn App enables contact tracing. If the person has contracted the virus and the information is loaded to the app, then when another user is within a distance of 2 m, it alerts the user by the exchange of coded messages between two phones, provided the app runs in the background of both the phones.

a) **Telemedicine**: Germany's health ministry and Docyet, a start-up firm, launched a chatbot to collect self-health information from people regarding their symptoms related to coronavirus. The chatbot app does analyse the user data and provides suggestions regarding their risk level and telemedicine choices from its database.

b) **Remote technology**: Blinkin an AI and AR-supported remote assistance technology which assists in setting up emergency medical infrastructure through teleportation of skills. The Blinkin is an Indo-German company that assisted hospitals in Wuhan, China and Huber & Ranner, an air-handling German company in installing the ventilation system, and air-handling units during COVID-19 pandemics. Blinkin is a software system that could run on a mobile phone powered with AI and AR-enabled intelligent eyes similar to a visual bot. The AI agents in the system analyse the location where installation setup is required and the AR system prompt augmented pointers and annotations. By this, the system guides the remote user with the necessary information.

e) **France**: A telephonic virtual voice assistance system 'AlloCovid' collects symptoms from the caller who has dialled the AlloCovid number. This system uses AI to interpret the speeches and based on the symptoms and pre-existing health conditions maps the caller to the appropriate healthcare professional. The system stores only the postal code of the caller to determine the cluster of COVID cases. This telemedicine system can receive 1000 calls simultaneously and reduce the burden on the emergency healthcare number. Further, it is convenient for people who wish to communicate over the phone, instead of through an app.

For instance, France government introduces 'stopcovid' a mobile app to trace contacts. When a person is diagnosed as corona infected, the hospital will provide a QR code. The patient has to upload it to the stopcovid app running on her phone to self-declare the illness. Since, the app collects the close contacts' information using Bluetooth during its operation, after the self-declaration, the ephemeral IDs of all close contacts collected by the app during the last 14 days will be trackable. Immediately, the system will map those ephemeral IDs to the people who had close contact with the person and alert them by sending them a notification [412].

Next, Paris metro used AI assistance to detect people not wearing the mask in metro stations. It uses AI software integrated into the surveillance cameras that could detect the people without the mask and generates some statistics for an interval of 15 minutes. These statistics help to determine the rate of an outbreak of COVID-19. The AI software developed by DatakaLab a start-up in Paris is lightweight meaning that the collected images are processed locally and are not stored in the cloud to protect the privacy of citizens [413].

11.4.1 UPDATES ON COVID-19 VACCINATIONS

After almost a year of hard grip on the entire world by COVID-19, recently, the world has started witnessing the launch of vaccinations. The vaccines produced by major organizations such as Pfizer, Moderna and Oxford University will witness a great challenge with regard to storage and distribution. This stems from the fact that the vaccines should be stored in an extreme temperature-controlled setting until they being used. For instance, Pfizer requires −70 deg. Celsius. Further, these vaccines should be transported in unprecedented volumes, at the earliest throughout the world. Next, the massive data log (gender, age, vaccine ID, the person who received the vaccination, date, and time etc.) of these vaccination processes has to be managed securely. The IoT is the best solution where sensors can monitor temperature, humidity, location and send this information to the delivery stations of the vaccine. In an instance, Controlant and Vodafone global IoT platform deployed their IoT solutions to monitor and track the vaccines in real time during shipment worldwide. The companies such as Romabee and Cloudleaf have extensively spent their resources to monitor the supply chain through passive GPS sensors [414]. HCL Technologies in India has used IoT for real-time location tracking and integrity management, blockchain-integrated custody management for detecting theft of vaccines during storage. Overall, in Figure 11.4, we have mentioned the key technologies that will find highly useful during storage, transport and data management of COVID-19 vaccination stages.

Moreover, several countries such as countries in Europe, China, India, Japan, etc., have issued digital vaccination passports to the citizens who already got vaccinated for COVID-19. It includes a digital copy of the vaccination details that shall be accessible through an app to allow international travel. For instance, India uses cowin.gov.in portal to register individuals for vaccination using phone verification.

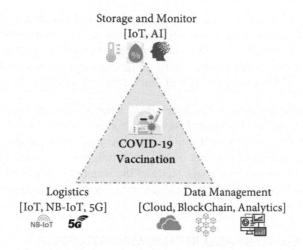

Figure 11.4 COVID-19 vaccination:assisting technologies

11.5   CHALLENGES IN IMPLEMENTATION

In this section, we briefly describe the key challenges in implementing smart health-care.

11.5.1   TECHNOLOGICAL CHALLENGES

i) Choice of technology: Various sectors of healthcare require different technolo-gies for their efficient operation. However, it is a big challenge to evaluate the full potential of a technology that suits the current requirements of smart healthcare. For instance, scaling from a medium-scale hospital to a large hos-pital should be easy with minimal burden on the existing connectivity, storage and computing facilities.

ii) Digital divide: While adopting new internet-based technologies such as telemedicine, remote robotic surgery, cloud-based AI solutions, 5G-IoT solu-tions in healthcare requires network connectivity as the primary requirement. Nevertheless, addressing the digital divide or poor network connectivity will become the primary concern of smart healthcare in rural areas.

iii) Security/privacy: Healthcare data is the most private information of an individ-ual. Consequently, while maintaining the privacy and security of patient data, cybercrimes and internet security threats are the key hurdles. In this regard, data privacy policies, intense research on blockchains and quantum comput-ing for internet security are foreseen.

11.5.2   SOCIETAL CHALLENGES

(i) Demographic factors/education: The patients of different age groups, gender, social background have non-uniform responses for smart healthcare. Due to this, the healthcare schemes have not reached effectively all sectors of soci-ety. Addressing this hurdle is also a big challenge to make smart healthcare inclusive. Moreover, poverty will also lead to inequality in smart healthcare.

(ii) Misconception about technology: There exist misconceptions about different ICT schemes used in smart healthcare. For instance, 5G is misunderstood as bad, mobile app for virtual consultation is considered to be least effective, etc. In addition, people may not provide the right data for studies due to fear of privacy breaches. A thorough study of the suitability of technology and inno-vative methods to overcome the inherent technological limitations is necessary.

11.6   DISCUSSIONS AND RECOMMENDATIONS

In this chapter, we highlighted the key technological solutions of different smart cities. The key observations have led us to the following discussions:

(i) Dubai has extensively used all its technical infrastructure to emerge as a hub of smart healthcare tourism. Following this, we observe Taipei, Singapore and Amsterdam's involvement in AI, robotics and IoT in healthcare has kept them ready to handle pandemics situations. For instance, Taiwan and Singapore are the best examples during COVID-19 to contain the spread of the virus.

(ii) Further, many smart cities are yet to integrate ICT in healthcare. Smart cities must set a balance between the resources sanctioned for smart healthcare and other components of the smart city project.

(iii) The Amsterdam and Tampere cities have balanced contribution to healthcare from industry, government, start-ups, universities when compared to other cities.

Based on our study, we have the following recommendations:

(i) Due to the exponential growth in the urban population, smart healthcare becomes inevitable to meet the healthcare challenges.

(ii) There is a need to develop more efficient smart solutions that would analyse the progress of epidemics and assist in the launch of suitable measures to contain future pandemic (COVID) situations.

(iii) The city governments must regulate access to personal health data to ascertain the privacy of individuals. Further, regulations regarding the safety of the use of 3D printed body parts, UAV and robotic surgery must be given the top priority in smart healthcare.

(iv) Further, based on the actions taken during COVID-19 outbreaks, we reckon that telemedicine and remote healthcare require tremendous attention with regard to ICT infrastructure across all small cities to equip the city authorities for better management of such situations.

References

1. H. Kalantarian, N. Alshurafa, and M. Sarrafzadeh, "A wearable nutrition monitoring system," in *11th IEEE International Conference on Wearable and Implantable Body Sensor Networks*, 2014, pp. 75–80.

2. F. Li, H. Wang, X. Shi, Y. Dai, and J. Zhang, "Direct patterning copper circuit on textile for wearable electronics," in *5th IEEE Electron Devices Technology & Manufacturing Conference (EDTM)*, 2021, pp. 1–3.

3. R. Narasimhan, T. Parlikar, G. Verghese, and M. V. McConnell, "Finger-wearable blood pressure monitor," in *40th Annual International Conference of the IEEE Engineering in Medicine and Biology Society (EMBC)*, 2018, pp. 3792–3795.

4. N. A. Choudhry, A. Rasheed, S. Ahmad, L. Arnold, and L. Wang, "Design, development and characterization of textile stitch-based piezoresistive sensors for wearable monitoring," *IEEE Sensors Journal*, vol. 20, no. 18, pp. 10485–10494, 2020.

5. V. V. Tipparaju, X. Xian, D. Bridgeman, D. Wang, F. Tsow, E. Forzani, and N. Tao, "Reliable breathing tracking with wearable mask device," *IEEE Sensors Journal*, vol. 20, no. 10, pp. 5510–5518, 2020.

6. H. Balasubramaniyam, M. Vignesh, A. Abhirami, A. Abanah *et al.*, "Design and development of a iot based flexible and wearable t-shirt for monitoring breathing rate," in *3rd IEEE International Conference on Computing Methodologies and Communication (ICCMC)*, 2019, pp. 376–379.

7. I. U. Ahmed, N. Hassan, and H. Rashid, "Solar powered smart wearable health monitoring and tracking device based on gps and gsm technology for children with autism," in *4th IEEE International Conference on Advances in Electrical Engineering (ICAEE)*, 2017, pp. 111–116.

8. G. Z. Yang and B. M. Rosa, "A wearable and battery-less device for assessing skin hydration level under direct sunlight exposure with ultraviolet index calculation," in *15th IEEE International Conference on Wearable and Implantable Body Sensor Networks (BSN)*, 2018, pp. 201–204.

9. A. Dinh, D. Teng, L. Chen, S.-B. Ko, Y. Shi, C. McCrosky, J. Basran, and V. Del Bello-Hass, "A wearable device for physical activity monitoring with built-in heart rate variability," in *3rd IEEE International Conference on Bioinformatics and Biomedical Engineering*, 2009, pp. 1–4.

10. W. A. Weeks, A. Dua, J. Hutchison, R. Joshi, R. Li, J. Szejer, and R. G. Azevedo, "A low-power, low-cost ingestible and wearable sensing platform to measure medication adherence and physiological signals," in *40th Annual International Conference of the IEEE Engineering in Medicine and Biology Society (EMBC)*, 2018, pp. 5549–5553.

11. A. Oliveira, D. Dias, E. M. Lopes, M. do Carmo Vilas-Boas, and J. P. S. Cunha, "A textile embedded wearable device for movement disorders quantification," in *42nd Annual International Conference of the IEEE Engineering in Medicine and Biology Society (EMBC)*, 2020, pp. 4559–4562.

12. R. Prasannan and G. Sarath, "Iot based device for fertility monitoring," in *5th IEEE International Conference on Communication and Electronics Systems (ICCES)*, 2020, pp. 813–817.

13. A. Bhuiyan, M. A. Islam, M. H. Shahriar, T. H. Supto, M. A. Kasem, and M. E. Daud, "An assistance system for visually challenged people based on computer vision and iot," in *IEEE Region 10 Symposium (TENSYMP)*, 2020, pp. 1359–1362.

14. D. L. Presti, C. Massaroni, J. Di Tocco, E. Schena, D. Formica, M. A. Caponero, U. G. Longo, A. Carnevale, J. D'Abbraccio, L. Massari *et al.*, "Cardiac monitoring with a smart textile based on polymer-encapsulated fbg: Influence of sensor positioning," in *IEEE International Symposium on Medical Measurements and Applications (MeMeA)*, 2019, pp. 1–6.

15. N. Sriraam, A. Srinivasulu, V. Prakash, and S. Sahoo, "A smart textile electrode belt for ecg recordings-a pilot study with indian population," in *2nd IEEE International Conference on Signal Processing and Communication (ICSPC)*, 2019, pp. 267–270.

16. I. M. Saied and T. Arslan, "Noninvasive wearable rf device towards monitoring brain atrophy and lateral ventricle enlargement," *IEEE Journal of Electromagnetics, RF and Microwaves in Medicine and Biology*, vol. 4, no. 1, pp. 61–68, 2019.

17. N. Kostikis, G. Rigas, N. Tachos, S. Konitsiotis, and D. I. Fotiadis, "On-body sensor position identification with a simple, robust and accurate method, validated in patients with parkinson's disease," in *42nd Annual International Conference of the IEEE Engineering in Medicine & Biology Society (EMBC)*, 2020, pp. 4156–4159.

18. U. D. L. Fadhillah, Z. A. N. Afikah, N. E. N. Safiee, A. W. Asnida, A. K. M. Rafiq, and M. H. Ramlee, "Development of a low-cost wearable breast cancer detection device," in *2nd IEEE International Conference on BioSignal Analysis, Processing and Systems (ICBAPS)*, 2018, pp. 41–46.

19. P. Sasidharan, T. Rajalakshmi, and U. Snekhalatha, "Wearable cardiorespiratory monitoring device for heart attack prediction," in *IEEE International Conference on Communication and Signal Processing (ICCSP)*, 2019, pp. 0054–0057.

20. Y. J. Jeon and S. J. Kang, "Wearable sleepcare kit: Analysis and prevention of sleep apnea symptoms in real-time," *IEEE Access*, vol. 7, pp. 60 634–60 649, 2019.

21. Z. G. Xiao and C. Menon, "Towards the development of a wearable feedback system for monitoring the activities of the upper-extremities," *Journal of Neuroengineering and Rehabilitation*, vol. 11, no. 1, pp. 1–13, 2014.

22. Y. Gu, T. Zhang, H. Chen, F. Wang, Y. Pu, C. Gao, and S. Li, "Mini review on flexible and wearable electronics for monitoring human health information," *Nanoscale Research Letters*, vol. 14, no. 1, pp. 1–15, 2019.

23. Z. U. Ahmed, M. G. Mortuza, M. J. Uddin, M. H. Kabir, M. Mahiuddin, and M. J. Hoque, "Internet of things based patient health monitoring system using wearable biomedical device," in *IEEE International Conference on Innovation in Engineering and Technology (ICIET)*, 2018, pp. 1–5.

24. O. Apilo, J. Mäkelä, and A. Kuosmonen, "Evaluation of cellular iot for sport wearables," in *IEEE 30th International Symposium on Personal, Indoor and Mobile Radio Communications (PIMRC Workshops)*, 2019, pp. 1–7.

25. J. M. Santos-Gago, M. Ramos-Merino, S. Vallarades-Rodriguez, L. M. Álvarez-Sabucedo, M. J. Fernández-Iglesias, and J. L. Garcia-Soidán, "Innovative use of wrist-worn wearable devices in the sports domain: A systematic review," *Electronics*, vol. 8, no. 11, p. 1257, 2019.

26. K. M. Diaz, D. J. Krupka, M. J. Chang, J. Peacock, Y. Ma, J. Goldsmith, J. E. Schwartz, and K. W. Davidson, "Fitbit: An accurate and reliable device for wireless physical activity tracking," *International Journal of Cardiology*, vol. 185, p. 138, 2015.

27. G. Aroganam, N. Manivannan, and D. Harrison, "Review on wearable technology sensors used in consumer sport applications," *Sensors*, vol. 19, no. 9, p. 1983, 2019.

28. V. Davies, E. M. Scott, M. L. Wiseman-Orr, A. K. Wright, and J. Reid, "Development of an early warning system for owners using a validated health-related quality of life (hrql) instrument for companion animals and its use in a large cohort of dogs," *Frontiers in Veterinary Science*, vol. 7, p. 652, 2020.

29. F. Cagnacci, L. Boitani, R. A. Powell, and M. S. Boyce, "Animal ecology meets gps-based radiotelemetry: A perfect storm of opportunities and challenges," 2010.

30. G. Di Gironimo, T. Caporaso, D. M. Del Giudice, and A. Lanzotti, "Towards a new monitoring system to detect illegal steps in race-walking," *International Journal on Interactive Design and Manufacturing (IJIDeM)*, vol. 11, no. 2, pp. 317–329, 2017.

31. J. Werner, L. Leso, C. Umstatter, M. Schick, B. O'Brien *et al.*, "Evaluation of precision technologies for measuring cows' grazing behaviour," *Grassland Resources for Extensive Farming Systems in Marginal Lands: Major Drivers and Future Scenarios*, vol. 82, 2017.

32. W. Gao, S. Emaminejad, H. Y. Y. Nyein, S. Challa, K. Chen, A. Peck, H. M. Fahad, H. Ota, H. Shiraki, D. Kiriya *et al.*, "Fully integrated wearable sensor arrays for multiplexed in situ perspiration analysis," *Nature*, vol. 529, no. 7587, pp. 509–514, 2016.

33. G. Pulkkis, J. Karlsson, M. Westerlund, and J. Tana, "Secure and reliable internet of things systems for healthcare," in *2017 IEEE 5th International Conference on Future Internet of Things and Cloud (FiCloud)*. IEEE, 2017, pp. 169–176.

34. T. Rifat, M. S. Hossain, M. M. Alam, and A. S. S. Rouf, "A review on applications of nanobots in combating complex diseases," *Bangladesh Pharmaceutical Journal*, vol. 22, no. 1, pp. 99–108, 2019.

35. I. R. Vanani and M. Amirhosseini, "Iot-based diseases prediction and diagnosis system for healthcare," in *Internet of Things for Healthcare Technologies*. Springer, 2021, pp. 21–48.

36. K. Byerly, L. Vagner, I. Grecu, G. Grecu, and G. Lazaroiu, "Real-time big data processing and wearable internet of medical things sensor devices for health monitoring," *American Journal of Medical Research*, vol. 6, no. 2, pp. 67–72, 2019.

37. S. Bhattacharya, "Patients satisfaction and role of phcs: A comparative study of two districts of north bengal," http://inet.vidyasagar.ac.in:8080/jspui/bitstream/123456789/1559/1/7.pdf, accessed: 2021-11-11.

38. S. Prabhu, C. Gooneratne, K. A. Hoang, and S. Mukhopadhyay, "Iot-associated impedimetric biosensing for point-of-care monitoring of kidney health," *IEEE Sensors Journal*, vol. 21, pp. 14320–14329, 2020.

39. J. Steurer, L. M. Bachmann, and O. S. Miettinen, "Etiology in a taxonomy of illnesses," *European Journal of Epidemiology*, vol. 21, no. 2, pp. 85–89, 2006.

40. I. F. Akyildiz, M. Ghovanloo, U. Guler, T. Ozkaya-Ahmadov, A. F. Sarioglu, and B. D. Unluturk, "Panacea: An internet of bio-nanothings application for early detection and mitigation of infectious diseases," *IEEE Access*, vol. 8, pp. 140 512–140 523, 2020.

41. D. L. Sackett, "Clinical epidemiology: What, who, and whither," *Journal of Clinical Epidemiology*, vol. 55, no. 12, pp. 1161–1166, 2002.

42. S. Ju, Y. Sun, and Y. Su, "Internet of things smart medical system and nursing intervention of glucocorticoid drug use," *Microprocessors and Microsystems*, vol. 83, p. 104008, 2021.

43. S. Cho, S. Jun, M. Lee, P.-s. Chung, S. Kim, B. Y. Hill, and B. J. Tromberg, "Rtbiot: A real-time healthcare monitoring bio-iot device employing spatially resolved near infrared (nir) spectroscopy," in *Optical Tomography and Spectroscopy of Tissue XIII*, vol. 10874. International Society for Optics and Photonics, 2019, p. 1087404.

44. R. Ani, S. Krishna, N. Anju, M. S. Aslam, and O. Deepa, "Iot based patient monitoring and diagnostic prediction tool using ensemble classifier," in *IEEE International Conference on Advances in Computing, Communications and Informatics (ICACCI)*, 2017, pp. 1588–1593.

45. P. Kumar, R. Chauhan, T. Stephan, A. Shankar, and S. Thakur, "A machine learning implementation for mental health care application: Smart watch for depression detection," in *11th IEEE International Conference on Cloud Computing, Data Science & Engineering (Confluence)*, 2021, pp. 568–574.

46. K. G. Moons, P. Royston, Y. Vergouwe, D. E. Grobbee, and D. G. Altman, "Prognosis and prognostic research: What, why, and how?" *BMJ*, vol. 338, 2009, Doi: 10.1136/bmj.b375.

47. Y. Uneno and M. Kanai, "Prognosis prediction models and their clinical utility in palliative care," *Highlights on Several Underestimated Topics in Palliative Care*, p. 129, 2017, DOI: 10.5772/intechopen.69663.

48. A. Tolba and Z. Al-Makhadmeh, "Wearable sensor-based fuzzy decision-making model for improving the prediction of human activities in rehabilitation," *Measurement*, vol. 166, p. 108254, 2020.

49. E. E. Holmes, "5. basic epidemiological concepts ina spatial context," in *Spatial Ecology*. Princeton University Press, 2018, pp. 111–136.

50. S. Kaushalya, K. Kulawansa, and M. Firdhous, "Internet of things for epidemic detection: A critical review," *Advances in Computer Communication and Computational Sciences*, vol. 924, pp. 485–495, 2019.

51. M. S. Shende and M. S. Hiray, "A prediction engine for influenza pandemic using healthcare analysis," *International Research Journal of Engineering and Technology (IRJET)*, pp. 3408–3410, 2018.

52. L. C. Harper, "2020 alzheimer's association facts and figures," https://www.cambridge.org/core/books/abs/tattoo-on-my-brain/resources/ 0792100A3FD2B91DE2B4CE89D2B0956B, accessed: 2021-11-11.

53. Z. H. K. Chong, Y. X. Tee, L. J. Toh, S. J. Phang, J. Y. Liew, B. Queck, and S. Gottipati, "Predicting potential alzheimer medical condition in elderly using iot sensors-case study," in *IEEE IRC Conference on Science, Engineering, and Technology*, 2017.

54. I. Ahmed, M. Ahmad, G. Jeon, and F. Piccialli, "A framework for pandemic prediction using big data analytics," *Big Data Research*, vol. 25, p. 100190, 2021.

55. S. S. Morse, J. A. Mazet, M. Woolhouse, C. R. Parrish, D. Carroll, W. B. Karesh, C. Zambrana-Torrelio, W. I. Lipkin, and P. Daszak, "Prediction and prevention of the next pandemic zoonosis," *The Lancet*, vol. 380, no. 9857, pp. 1956–1965, 2012.

56. H. D. Marston, C. I. Paules, and A. S. Fauci, "The critical role of biomedical research in pandemic preparedness," *Jama*, vol. 318, no. 18, pp. 1757–1758, 2017.

57. V. S. Rohila, N. Gupta, A. Kaul, and D. K. Sharma, "Deep learning assisted covid-19 detection using full ct-scans," *Internet of Things*, vol. 14, p. 100377, 2021.

58. B. Muthu, C. Sivaparthipan, G. Manogaran, R. Sundarasekar, S. Kadry, A. Shanthini, and A. Dasel, "Iot based wearable sensor for diseases prediction and symptom analysis in healthcare sector," *Peer-to-peer Networking and Applications*, vol. 13, no. 6, pp. 2123–2134, 2020.

59. R. S. Istepanian, S. Hu, N. Y. Philip, and A. Sungoor, "The potential of internet of m-health things "m-iot" for non-invasive glucose level sensing," in *Annual International Conference of the IEEE Engineering in Medicine and Biology Society*, 2011, pp. 5264–5266.

60. A. Avinashiappan and B. Mayilsamy, "Internet of medical things: Security threats, security challenges, and potential solutions," *Internet of Medical Things: Remote Healthcare Systems and Applications*, p. 1, 2021.

61. G. Rathee, A. Sharma, H. Saini, R. Kumar, and R. Iqbal, "A hybrid framework for multimedia data processing in iot-healthcare using blockchain technology," *Multimedia Tools and Applications*, vol. 79, no. 15, pp. 9711–9733, 2020.

62. W. Zhuang, Y. Chen, J. Su, B. Wang, and C. Gao, "Design of human activity recognition algorithms based on a single wearable imu sensor," *International Journal of Sensor Networks*, vol. 30, no. 3, pp. 193–206, 2019.

63. A. Manzi, F. Cavallo, and P. Dario, "A neural network approach to human posture classification and fall detection using rgb-d camera," in *Italian Forum of Ambient Assisted Living*. Springer, 2016, pp. 127–139.

64. P. Rosero-Montalvo, D. Jaramillo, S. Flores, D. Peluffo, V. Alvear, and M. Lopez, "Human sit down position detection using data classification and dimensionality reduction," *Advances in Science, Technology and Engineering Systems Journal*, vol. 2, no. 3, pp. 749–754, 2017.

65. K. Arora, P. Gupta, S. Chopra, and N. Pathak, "Posture monitoring belt," *International Journal of Innovation Research Studies*, vol. 4, pp. 150–159, 2015.

66. T. Hussain, H. F. Maqbool, N. Iqbal, M. Khan, Salman, and A. A. Dehghani-Sanij, "Computational model for the recognition of lower limb movement using wearable gyroscope sensor," *International Journal of Sensor Networks*, vol. 30, no. 1, pp. 35–45, 2019.

67. Q. Wang, W. Chen, A. A. Timmermans, C. Karachristos, J.-B. Martens, and P. Markopoulos, "Smart rehabilitation garment for posture monitoring," in *37th Annual International Conference of the IEEE Engineering in Medicine and Biology Society (EMBC)*, 2015, pp. 5736–5739.

68. C. Lim, S. Basah, M. Ali, and C. Fook, "Wearable posture identification system for good sitting position," *Journal of Telecommunication, Electronic and Computer Engineering (JTEC)*, vol. 10, no. 1-16, pp. 135–140, 2018.

69. E. Farella, A. Pieracci, L. Benini, and A. Acquaviva, "A wireless body area sensor network for posture detection," in *11th IEEE Symposium on Computers and Communications (ISCC'06)*, 2006, pp. 454–459.

70. E. Farella, A. Pieracci, and A. Acquaviva, "Design and implementation of wimoca node for a body area wireless sensor network," in *IEEE Systems Communications (ICW'05, ICHSN'05, ICMCS'05, SENET'05)*, 2005, pp. 342–347.

71. R. Alattas and K. M. Elleithy, "Detecting bad posture using postuino among engineering graduate students," 2015.

72. J. A. Walraven *et al.*, "Introduction to applications and industries for microelectromechanical systems (mems)." in *ITC*, 2003, pp. 674–680.

73. N. Instruments, "Strain gauge measurement–a tutorial," 1998.

74. A. Y. Tang, C.-H. Ong, and A. Ahmad, "Fall detection sensor system for the elderly," *International Journal of Advanced Computer Research*, vol. 5, no. 19, p. 176, 2015.

75. F. Wu, H. Zhao, Y. Zhao, and H. Zhong, "Development of a wearable-sensor-based fall detection system," *International Journal of Telemedicine and Applications*, vol. 2015, pp. 1–11, 2015.

76. S. Chaudhuri, H. Thompson, and G. Demiris, "Fall detection devices and their use with older adults: A systematic review," *Journal of Geriatric Physical Therapy (2001)*, vol. 37, no. 4, p. 178, 2014.

77. X. Wang, J. Ellul, and G. Azzopardi, "Elderly fall detection systems: A literature survey," *Frontiers in Robotics AI*, vol. 7, p. 71, 2020.

78. P. Vallabh and R. Malekian, "Fall detection monitoring systems: A comprehensive review," *Journal of Ambient Intelligence and Humanized Computing*, vol. 9, no. 6, pp. 1809–1833, 2018.

79. K.-D. Chang, C.-Y. Chen, J.-L. Chen, and H.-C. Chao, "Internet of things and cloud computing for future internet," in *International Conference on Securityenriched Urban Computing and Smart Grid.* Springer, 2011, pp. 1–10.

80. B. S. Babu, K. Srikanth, T. Ramanjaneyulu, and I. L. Narayana, "Iot for healthcare," *International Journal of Science and Research*, vol. 5, no. 2, pp. 322–326, 2016.

81. "Arduino home," $https://www.arduino.cc/$, accessed: 2021-08-11.

82. "Raspberry pi," https://www.raspberrypi.org/, accessed: 2021-08-11.

83. K.-H. Chang, "Bluetooth: A viable solution for iot?[industry perspectives]," *IEEE Wireless Communications*, vol. 21, no. 6, pp. 6–7, 2014.

84. C. Shi, J. Liu, H. Liu, and Y. Chen, "Smart user authentication through actuation of daily activities leveraging wifi-enabled iot," in *Proceedings of the 18th ACM International Symposium on Mobile Ad Hoc Networking and Computing*, 2017, pp. 1–10.

85. S. M. Fati, A. Muneer, D. Mungur, and A. Badawi, "Integrated health monitoring system using gsm and iot," in *IEEE International Conference on Smart Computing and Electronic Enterprise (ICSCEE)*, 2018, pp. 1–7.

86. Y. Yuehong, Y. Zeng, X. Chen, and Y. Fan, "The internet of things in healthcare: An overview," *Journal of Industrial Information Integration*, vol. 1, pp. 3–13, 2016.

87. J.-S. Wang, W.-C. Chiang, Y.-L. Hsu, and Y.-T. C. Yang, "Ecg arrhythmia classification using a probabilistic neural network with a feature reduction method," *Neurocomputing*, vol. 116, pp. 38–45, 2013.

88. C. Hu, R. Ju, Y. Shen, P. Zhou, and Q. Li, "Clinical decision support for alzheimer's disease based on deep learning and brain network," in *IEEE International Conference on Communications (ICC)*, 2016, pp. 1–6.

89. S. Khalid, A. Judge, and R. Pinedo-Villanueva, "An unsupervised learning model for pattern recognition in routinely collected healthcare data," pp. 1–8, 2018.

90. X. Wang, D. Sontag, and F. Wang, "Unsupervised learning of disease progression models," in *Proceedings of the 20th ACM SIGKDD International Conference on Knowledge Discovery and Data Mining*, 2014, pp. 85–94.

91. G. Zhang, S.-X. Ou, Y.-H. Huang, and C.-R. Wang, "Semi-supervised learning methods for large scale healthcare data analysis," *International Journal of Computers in Healthcare*, vol. 2, no. 2, pp. 98–110, 2015.

92. R. Rezvani, S. Kouchaki, R. Nilforooshan, D. J. Sharp, and P. Barnaghi, "Semi-supervised learning for identifying the likelihood of agitation in people with dementia," *arXiv preprint arXiv:2105.10398*, 2021.

93. Y. Chen, X. Qin, J. Wang, C. Yu, and W. Gao, "Fedhealth: A federated transfer learning framework for wearable healthcare," *IEEE Intelligent Systems*, vol. 35, no. 4, pp. 83–93, 2020.

94. A. Alghamdi, M. Hammad, H. Ugail, A. Abdel-Raheem, K. Muhammad, H. S. Khalifa, and A. A. A. El-Latif, "Detection of myocardial infarction based on novel deep transfer learning methods for urban healthcare in smart cities," *arXiv preprint arXiv:1906.09358*, 2019.

95. I. Steinwart and A. Christmann, *Support Vector Machines*. Springer Science & Business Media, 2008.

96. N. Koutsouleris, E. M. Meisenzahl, C. Davatzikos, R. Bottlender, T. Frodl, J. Scheuerecker, G. Schmitt, T. Zetzsche, P. Decker, M. Reiser *et al.*, "Use of neuroanatomical pattern classification to identify subjects in at-risk mental states of psychosis and predict disease transition," *Archives of General Psychiatry*, vol. 66, no. 7, pp. 700–712, 2009.

97. S. Patel, K. Lorincz, R. Hughes, N. Huggins, J. Growdon, D. Standaert, M. Akay, J. Dy, M. Welsh, and P. Bonato, "Monitoring motor fluctuations in patients with parkinson's disease using wearable sensors," *IEEE Transactions on Information Technology in Biomedicine*, vol. 13, no. 6, pp. 864–873, 2009.

98. M. Bsoul, H. Minn, and L. Tamil, "Apnea medassist: Real-time sleep apnea monitor using single-lead ecg," *IEEE Transactions on Information Technology in Biomedicine*, vol. 15, no. 3, pp. 416–427, 2010.

99. A. Sano and R. W. Picard, "Stress recognition using wearable sensors and mobile phones," in *IEEE Humaine Association Conference on Affective Computing and Intelligent Interaction*, 2013, pp. 671–676.

100. L. B. Leng, L. B. Giin, and W.-Y. Chung, "Wearable driver drowsiness detection system based on biomedical and motion sensors," in *2015 IEEE SENSORS*. IEEE, 2015, pp. 1–4.

101. D. J. Hand and K. Yu, "Idiot's bayes—not so stupid after all?" *International Statistical Review*, vol. 69, no. 3, pp. 385–398, 2001.

102. J. Wijsman, B. Grundlehner, H. Liu, H. Hermens, and J. Penders, "Towards mental stress detection using wearable physiological sensors," in *Annual International Conference of the IEEE Engineering in Medicine and Biology Society*, 2011, pp. 1798–1801.

103. A. Gruenerbl, V. Osmani, G. Bahle, J. C. Carrasco, S. Oehler, O. Mayora, C. Haring, and P. Lukowicz, "Using smart phone mobility traces for the diagnosis of depressive and manic episodes in bipolar patients," in *Proceedings of the 5th Augmented Human International Conference*, 2014, pp. 1–8.

104. A. Grünerbl, A. Muaremi, V. Osmani, G. Bahle, S. Oehler, G. Tröster, O. Mayora, C. Haring, and P. Lukowicz, "Smartphone-based recognition of states and state changes in bipolar disorder patients," *IEEE Journal of Biomedical and Health Informatics*, vol. 19, no. 1, pp. 140–148, 2014.

105. E. Garcia-Ceja, V. Osmani, and O. Mayora, "Automatic stress detection in working environments from smartphones' accelerometer data: A first step," *IEEE Journal of Biomedical and Health Informatics*, vol. 20, no. 4, pp. 1053–1060, 2015.

106. N. S. Altman, "An introduction to kernel and nearest-neighbor nonparametric regression," *The American Statistician*, vol. 46, no. 3, pp. 175–185, 1992.

107. T. Lan, A. Adami, D. Erdogmus, and M. Pavel, "Estimating cognitive state using eeg signals," in *13th IEEE European Signal Processing Conference*, 2005, pp. 1–4.

108. H. Ghasemzadeh, N. Amini, R. Saeedi, and M. Sarrafzadeh, "Power-aware computing in wearable sensor networks: An optimal feature selection," *IEEE Transactions on Mobile Computing*, vol. 14, no. 4, pp. 800–812, 2014.

109. T. T. Ngo, Y. Makihara, H. Nagahara, Y. Mukaigawa, and Y. Yagi, "Similar gait action recognition using an inertial sensor," *Pattern Recognition*, vol. 48, no. 4, pp. 1289–1301, 2015.

110. J. J. Hopfield, "Artificial neural networks," *IEEE Circuits and Devices Magazine*, vol. 4, no. 5, pp. 3–10, 1988.

111. D. Wu, K. Warwick, Z. Ma, M. N. Gasson, J. G. Burgess, S. Pan, and T. Z. Aziz, "Prediction of parkinson's disease tremor onset using a radial basis function neural network based on particle swarm optimization," *International Journal of Neural Systems*, vol. 20, no. 02, pp. 109–116, 2010.

112. A. Krizhevsky, I. Sutskever, and G. E. Hinton, "Imagenet classification with deep convolutional neural networks," *Advances in Neural Information Processing Systems*, vol. 25, pp. 1097–1105, 2012.

113. Y. Zhang, Y. Sun, P. Phillips, G. Liu, X. Zhou, and S. Wang, "A multilayer perceptron based smart pathological brain detection system by fractional fourier entropy," *Journal of Medical Systems*, vol. 40, no. 7, pp. 1–11, 2016.

114. Z. Zhang, F. Ringeval, J. Han, J. Deng, E. Marchi, and B. Schuller, "Facing realism in spontaneous emotion recognition from speech: Feature enhancement by autoencoder with lstm neural networks," in *Proceedings INTERSPEECH 2016, 17th Annual Conference of the International Speech Communication Association (ISCA)*, 2016, pp. 3593–3597.

115. S. B. Hu, D. J. Wong, A. Correa, N. Li, and J. C. Deng, "Prediction of clinical deterioration in hospitalized adult patients with hematologic malignancies using a neural network model," *PloS One*, vol. 11, no. 8, p. e0161401, 2016.

116. M. G. Ruano, E. Hajimani, and A. Ruano, "A radial basis function classifier for the automatic diagnosis of cerebral vascular accidents," in *IEEE Global Medical Engineering Physics Exchanges/Pan American Health Care Exchanges (GMEPE/PAHCE)*, 2016, pp. 1–4.

117. H. Chen, X. Qi, L. Yu, and P.-A. Heng, "Dcan: Deep contour-aware networks for accurate gland segmentation," in *Proceedings of the IEEE Conference on Computer Vision and Pattern Recognition*, 2016, pp. 2487–2496.

118. W. Huang, C. P. Bridge, J. A. Noble, and A. Zisserman, "Temporal heartnet: Towards human-level automatic analysis of fetal cardiac screening video," in *International Conference on Medical Image Computing and Computer-Assisted Intervention*. Springer, 2017, pp. 341–349.

119. S. Wang, S. Du, Y. Li, H. Lu, M. Yang, B. Liu, and Y. Zhang, "Hearing loss detection in medical multimedia data by discrete wavelet packet entropy and single-hidden layer neural network trained by adaptive learning-rate back propagation," in *International Symposium on Neural Networks*. Springer, 2017, pp. 541–549.

120. J. D. Young, C. Cai, and X. Lu, "Unsupervised deep learning reveals prognostically relevant subtypes of glioblastoma," *BMC Bioinformatics*, vol. 18, no. 11, pp. 5–17, 2017.

121. M. Gao, Z. Xu, L. Lu, A. P. Harrison, R. M. Summers, and D. J. Mollura, "Holistic interstitial lung disease detection using deep convolutional neural networks: Multi-label learning and unordered pooling," *arXiv preprint arXiv:1701.05616*, 2017.

122. R. Salvador, S. Ortega, D. Madroñal, H. Fabelo, R. Lazcano, G. Marrero, E. Juárez, R. Sarmiento, and C. Sanz, "Helicoid: Interdisciplinary and collaborative project for real-time brain cancer detection," in *Proceedings of the Computing Frontiers Conference*, 2017, pp. 313–318.

123. I. M. Baytas, C. Xiao, X. Zhang, F. Wang, A. K. Jain, and J. Zhou, "Patient subtyping via time-aware lstm networks," in *Proceedings of the 23rd ACM SIGKDD International Conference on Knowledge Discovery and Data Mining*, 2017, pp. 65–74.

124. P. Rajpurkar, A. Y. Hannun, M. Haghpanahi, C. Bourn, and A. Y. Ng, "Cardiologist-level arrhythmia detection with convolutional neural networks," *arXiv preprint arXiv:1707.01836*, 2017.

125. O. Deperlioglu, U. Kose, D. Gupta, A. Khanna, and A. K. Sangaiah, "Diagnosis of heart diseases by a secure internet of health things system based on autoencoder deep neural network," *Computer Communications*, vol. 162, pp. 31–50, 2020.

126. S. Adhikary, S. Chaturvedi, S. K. Chaturvedi, and S. Banerjee, "Covid-19 spreading prediction and impact analysis by using artificial intelligence for sustainable global health assessment," in *Advances in Environment Engineering and Management*. Springer, 2021, pp. 375–386.

127. M. Abdel-Basset, H. Hawash, R. K. Chakrabortty, M. Ryan, M. Elhoseny, and H. Song, "St-deephar: Deep learning model for human activity recognition in ioht applications," *IEEE Internet of Things Journal*, vol. 8, no. 6, pp. 4969–4979, 2020.

128. A. Khamparia, D. Gupta, V. H. C. de Albuquerque, A. K. Sangaiah, and R. H. Jhaveri, "Internet of health things-driven deep learning system for detection and classification of cervical cells using transfer learning," *The Journal of Supercomputing*, pp. 1–19, 2020.

129. E. A. Keshner and A. Lamontagne, "The untapped potential of virtual reality in rehabilitation of balance and gait in neurological disorders," *Frontiers in Virtual Reality*, vol. 2, p. 6, 2021.

130. S. Chakraborty, T. Suzuki, A. Das, A. Nandy, and G. Venture, "Gait abnormality detection using deep convolution network," in *Handbook of Research on Engineering, Business, and Healthcare Applications of Data Science and Analytics*. IGI Global, 2021, pp. 363–372.

131. S. Fujiwara, S. Sato, A. Sugawara, Y. Nishikawa, T. Koji, Y. Nishimura, and K. Ogasawara, "The coefficient of variation of step time can overestimate gait abnormality: Test-retest reliability of gait-related parameters obtained with a tri-axial accelerometer in healthy subjects," *Sensors*, vol. 20, no. 3, p. 577, 2020.

132. A. Michelini, A. Eshraghi, and J. Andrysek, "Two-dimensional video gait analysis: A systematic review of reliability, validity, and best practice considerations," *Prosthetics and Orthotics International*, vol. 44, no. 4, pp. 245–262, 2020.

133. M. Lee, C. Youm, B. Noh, and H. Park, "Gait characteristics based on shoe-type inertial measurement units in healthy young adults during treadmill walking," *Sensors*, vol. 20, no. 7, 2020. [Online]. Available: https://www.mdpi.com/1424-8220/20/7/2095

134. S. Adhikary, R. Ghosh, and A. Ghosh, "Gait abnormality detection without clinical intervention using wearable sensors and machine learning," in *Innovations in Sustainable Energy and Technology*. Springer, 2021, pp. 359–368.

135. Y. Zheng, Y. Weng, X. Yang, G. Cai, G. Cai, and Y. Song, "Svm-based gait analysis and classification for patients with parkinson's disease," in *2021 15th International Symposium on Medical Information and Communication Technology (ISMICT)*, 2021, pp. 53–58.

136. H. Arshad, M. A. Khan, M. I. Sharif, M. Yasmin, J. M. R. Tavares, Y.-D. Zhang, and S. C. Satapathy, "A multilevel paradigm for deep convolutional neural network features selection with an application to human gait recognition," *Expert Systems*, p. e12541, 2020.

137. Z. Zhang, T. He, M. Zhu, Z. Sun, Q. Shi, J. Zhu, B. Dong, M. R. Yuce, and C. Lee, "Deep learning-enabled triboelectric smart socks for iot-based gait analysis and vr applications," *NPJ Flexible Electronics*, vol. 4, no. 1, pp. 1–12, 2020.

138. C. Stergiou, K. E. Psannis, B. B. Gupta, and Y. Ishibashi, "Security, privacy & efficiency of sustainable cloud computing for big data & iot," *Sustainable Computing: Informatics and Systems*, vol. 19, pp. 174–184, 2018.

139. A. Datta, V. Bhatia, J. Noll, and S. Dixit, "Bridging the digital divide: Challenges in opening the digital world to the elderly, poor, and digitally illiterate," *IEEE Consumer Electronics Magazine*, vol. 8, no. 1, pp. 78–81, 2018.

140. F. Kammüller, O. O. Ogunyanwo, and C. W. Probst, "Designing data protection for gdpr compliance into iot healthcare systems," *arXiv preprint arXiv:1901.02426*, 2019.

141. P. Schulz, M. Matthe, H. Klessig, M. Simsek, G. Fettweis, J. Ansari, S. A. Ashraf, B. Almeroth, J. Voigt, I. Riedel *et al.*, "Latency critical iot applications in 5g: Perspective on the design of radio interface and network architecture," *IEEE Communications Magazine*, vol. 55, no. 2, pp. 70–78, 2017.

142. Y. H. Hwang, "Iot security & privacy: Threats and challenges," in *Proceedings of the 1st ACM Workshop on IoT Privacy, Trust, and Security*, 2015, pp. 1–1.

143. D. Arellanes and K.-K. Lau, "Evaluating iot service composition mechanisms for the scalability of iot systems," *Future Generation Computer Systems*, vol. 108, pp. 827–848, 2020.

144. T. Perković, S. Damjanović, P. Šolić, L. Patrono, and J. J. Rodrigues, "Meeting challenges in iot: Sensing, energy efficiency, and the implementation," in *Fourth International Congress on Information and Communication Technology*. Springer, 2020, pp. 419–430.

145. K. A. Darabkh, K. K. Wafa'a, and K. Ala'F, "Maximizing the life time of wireless sensor networks over iot environment," in *2020 Fifth International Conference on Fog and Mobile Edge Computing (FMEC)*. IEEE, 2020, pp. 270–274.

146. Forbes, "How many things are currently connected to the "internet of things" (iot)?" https://www.forbes.com/sites/quora/2013/01/07/how-many-things-are-currently-connected-to-the-internet-of-\things-iot/#20903a3ebd2d, accessed: 2021-11-11.

147. S. S. Srivastava, N. Gupta, and R. Jaiswal, "Modified version of playfair cipher by using 8x8 matrix and random number generation," in *IEEE 3rd International Conference on Computer Modeling and Simulatio*, 2011.

148. D. Evans, "The internet of things how the next evolution of the internet is changing everything," http://www.cisco.com/c/dam/en˙us/about/ac79/docs/innov/IoT˙IBSG˙0411FINAL.pdf, accessed: 2021-11-11.

149. L. Atzori, A. Iera, and G. Morabito, "The internet of things: A survey," *Computer Networks*, vol. 54, no. 15, pp. 2787–2805, 2010.

150. A. Al-Fuqaha, M. Guizani, M. Mohammadi, M. Aledhari, and M. Ayyash, "Internet of things: A survey on enabling technologies, protocols, and applications," *IEEE Communications Surveys & Tutorials*, vol. 17, no. 4, pp. 2347–2376, 2015.

151. A. Gluhak, S. Krco, M. Nati, D. Pfisterer, N. Mitton, and T. Razafindralambo, "A survey on facilities for experimental internet of things research," *IEEE Communications Magazine*, vol. 49, no. 11, pp. 58–67, 2011.

152. P. Gope, Y. Gheraibia, S. Kabir, and B. Sikdar, "A secure iot-based modern healthcare system with fault-tolerant decision making process," *IEEE Journal of Biomedical and Health Informatics*, vol. 25, no. 3, pp. 862–873, 2021.

153. L. Greco, G. Percannella, P. Ritrovato, F. Tortorella, and M. Vento, "Trends in iot based solutions for health care: Moving ai to the edge," *Pattern Recognition Letters*, vol. 135, pp. 346–353, 2020. [Online]. Available: https://www.sciencedirect.com/science/article/pii/S0167865520301884

154. F. T. Al-Dhief, N. M. A. Latiff, N. N. N. A. Malik, N. S. Salim, M. M. Baki, M. A. A. Albadr, and M. A. Mohammed, "A survey of voice pathology surveillance systems based on internet of things and machine learning algorithms," *IEEE Access*, vol. 8, pp. 64 514–64 533, 2020.

155. P. López, D. Fernández, A. J. Jara, and A. F. Skarmeta, "Survey of internet of things technologies for clinical environments," in *27th IEEE International Conference on Advanced Information Networking and Applications Workshops*, 2013, pp. 1349–1354.

156. S. M. R. Islam, D. Kwak, H. Kabir, M. Hossain, and K. Kwak, "The internet of things for health care : A comprehensive survey," *Access IEEE*, vol. 3, pp. 678–708, 2015.

157. S. Durga, R. Nag, and E. Daniel, "Survey on machine learning and deep learning algorithms used in internet of things (iot) healthcare," in *2019 3rd International Conference on Computing Methodologies and Communication (ICCMC)*, 2019, pp. 1018–1022.

158. M. Haghi, S. Neubert, A. Geissler, H. Fleischer, N. Stoll, R. Stoll, and K. Thurow, "A flexible and pervasive iot-based healthcare platform for physiological and environmental parameters monitoring," *IEEE Internet of Things Journal*, vol. 7, no. 6, pp. 5628–5647, 2020.

159. P. Langley and H. A. Simon, "Applications of machine learning and rule induction," vol. 38, no. 11, 1995. [Online]. Available: https://doi.org/10.1145/219717.219768

160. L. Breiman, "Statistical Modeling: The Two Cultures (with comments and a rejoinder by the author)," *Statistical Science*, vol. 16, no. 3, pp. 199 – 231, 2001. [Online]. Available: https://doi.org/10.1214/ss/1009213726

161. R. M. Hoogeveen, J. P. B. Pereira, N. S. Nurmohamed, V. Zampoleri, M. J. Bom, A. Baragetti, S. M. Boekholdt, P. Knaapen, K.-T. Khaw, N. J. Wareham *et al.*, "Improved cardiovascular risk prediction using targeted plasma proteomics in primary prevention," *European Heart Journal*, vol. 41, no. 41, pp. 3998–4007, 2020.

162. I. d. M. B. Filho, G. Aquino, R. S. Malaquias, G. Girão, and S. R. M. Melo, "An iot-based healthcare platform for patients in icu beds during the covid-19 outbreak," *IEEE Access*, vol. 9, pp. 27262–27277, 2021.

163. E. G. Ross, N. H. Shah, R. L. Dalman, K. T. Nead, J. P. Cooke, and N. J. Leeper, "The use of machine learning for the identification of peripheral artery disease and future mortality risk," *Journal of Vascular Surgery*, vol. 64, no. 5, pp. 1515–1522, 2016.

164. D. W. Bates, S. Saria, L. Ohno-Machado, A. Shah, and G. Escobar, "Big data in health care: Using analytics to identify and manage high-risk and high-cost patients," *Health Affairs*, vol. 33, no. 7, pp. 1123–1131, 2014.

165. V. Tiwari, W. R. Furman, and W. S. Sandberg, "Predicting case volume from the accumulating elective operating room schedule facilitates staffing improvements," *Anesthesiology*, vol. 121, no. 1, pp. 171–183, 2014.

166. J. S. Peck, J. C. Benneyan, D. J. Nightingale, and S. A. Gaehde, "Predicting emergency department inpatient admissions to improve same-day patient flow," *Academic Emergency Medicine*, vol. 19, no. 9, pp. E1045–E1054, 2012.

167. S. D. Fihn, J. Francis, C. Clancy, C. Nielson, K. Nelson, J. Rumsfeld, T. Cullen, J. Bates, and G. L. Graham, "Insights from advanced analytics at the veterans health administration," *Health Affairs*, vol. 33, no. 7, pp. 1203–1211, 2014.

168. S. Kumar, R. D. Raut, and B. E. Narkhede, "A proposed collaborative framework by using artificial intelligence-internet of things (ai-iot) in covid-19 pandemic situation for healthcare workers," *International Journal of Healthcare Management*, vol. 13, no. 4, pp. 337–345, 2020.

169. R. P. Singh, M. Javaid, A. Haleem, R. Vaishya, and S. Ali, "Internet of medical things (iomt) for orthopaedic in covid-19 pandemic: Roles, challenges, and applications," *Journal of Clinical Orthopaedics and Trauma*, vol. 11, no. 4, pp. 713–717, 2020.

170. A. A. Mawgoud, A. El Karadawy, and B. Tawfik, "A secure authentication technique in internet of medical things through machine learning," 12 2019.

171. F. Firouzi, B. Farahani, M. Ibrahim, and K. Chakrabarty, "Keynote paper: From eda to iot ehealth: Promises, challenges, and solutions," *IEEE Transactions on Computer-Aided Design of Integrated Circuits and Systems*, vol. 37, no. 12, pp. 2965–2978, 2018.

172. L. M. R. Tarouco, L. M. Bertholdo, L. Z. Granville, L. M. R. Arbiza, F. Carbone, M. Marotta, and J. J. C. De Santanna, "Internet of things in healthcare: Interoperatibility and security issues," in *IEEE International Conference on Communications (ICC)*, 2012, pp. 6121–6125.

173. M. intelligence, "Internet of medical things (iomt) market - growth, trends, covid-19 impact, and forcasts (2021–2026)," https://www.mordorintelligence.com/industry-reports/internet-of-medical-things-market, accessed: 2021-10-11.

174. S. R. Department, "Projected size of the internet of things (iot) in healthcare market worldwide from 2016 to 2025 (in billion u.s. dollars)," https://www.statista.com/statistics/997959/worldwide-internet-of-things-in-healthcare-market-size/, accessed: 2021-11-11.

175. S. S. Sarmah, "An efficient iot-based patient monitoring and heart disease prediction system using deep learning modified neural network," *IEEE Access*, vol. 8, pp. 135784–135797, 2020.

176. K. Darshan and K. Anandakumar, "A comprehensive review on usage of internet of things (iot) in healthcare system," in *2015 International Conference on Emerging Research in Electronics, Computer Science and Technology (ICERECT)*. IEEE, 2015, pp. 132–136.

177. A. S. Yeole and D. R. Kalbande, "Use of internet of things (iot) in healthcare: A survey," in *Proceedings of the ACM Symposium on Women in Research 2016*, 2016, pp. 71–76.

178. A. H. A. editorial staff, "Implatable medical devices," https://www.heart.org/en/health-topics/heart-attack/treatment-of-a-heart-attack/implantable-medical-devices, accessed: 2021-9-11.

179. N. A. Spaan, A. E. Teplova, E. Renard, and J. A. Spaan, "Implantable insulin pumps: An effective option with restricted dissemination," *The Lancet Diabetes & Endocrinology*, vol. 2, no. 5, pp. 358–360, 2014.

180. R. K. Kodali, G. Swamy, and B. Lakshmi, "An implementation of iot for healthcare," in *2015 IEEE Recent Advances in Intelligent Computational Systems (RAICS)*. IEEE, 2015, pp. 411–416.

181. R. Somasundaram and M. Thirugnanam, "Review of security challenges in healthcare internet of things," *Wireless Networks*, vol. 27, no. 8, pp. 5503–5509, 2021.

182. M. N. Alraja, M. M. J. Farooque, and B. Khashab, "The effect of security, privacy, familiarity, and trust on users' attitudes toward the use of the iot-based healthcare: The mediation role of risk perception," *IEEE Access*, vol. 7, pp. 111 341–111 354, 2019.

183. L. O'Donnell, "More than half of iot devices vulnerable to severe attacks," https://threatpost.com/half-iot-devices-vulnerable-severe-attacks/153609/., accessed: 2021-9-21.

184. Y. Sun, F. P.-W. Lo, and B. Lo, "Security and privacy for the internet of medical things enabled healthcare systems: A survey," *IEEE Access*, vol. 7, pp. 183 339–183 355, 2019.

185. M. Papaioannou, M. Karageorgou, G. Mantas, V. Sucasas, I. Essop, J. Rodriguez, and D. Lymberopoulos, "A survey on security threats and countermeasures in internet of medical things (iomt)," *Transactions on Emerging Telecommunications Technologies*, p. e4049, 2020.

186. A. M. Altamimi *et al.*, "Security and privacy issues in ehealthcare systems: Towards trusted services," *International Journal of Advanced Computer Science and Applications*, vol. 7, no. 9, pp. 229–236, 2016.

187. S. Pundir, M. Wazid, D. P. Singh, A. K. Das, J. J. Rodrigues, and Y. Park, "Intrusion detection protocols in wireless sensor networks integrated to internet of things deployment: Survey and future challenges," *IEEE Access*, vol. 8, pp. 3343–3363, 2019.

188. R. Saeedi, J. Purath, K. Venkatasubramanian, and H. Ghasemzadeh, "Toward seamless wearable sensing: Automatic on-body sensor localization for physical activity monitoring," in *36th Annual International Conference of the IEEE Engineering in Medicine and Biology Society*, 2014, pp. 5385–5388.

189. J. Y. Kim, W. Hu, H. Shafagh, and S. Jha, "Seda: Secure over-the-air code dissemination protocol for the internet of things," *IEEE Transactions on Dependable and Secure Computing*, vol. 15, no. 6, pp. 1041–1054, 2016.

190. R. Boussada, B. Hamdane, M. E. Elhdhili, and L. A. Saidane, "Privacy-preserving aware data transmission for iot-based e-health," *Computer Networks*, vol. 162, p. 106866, 2019.

191. M. Wazid, A. K. Das, J. J. Rodrigues, S. Shetty, and Y. Park, "Iomt malware detection approaches: Analysis and research challenges," *IEEE Access*, vol. 7, pp. 182 459–182 476, 2019.

192. V. Alagar, A. Alsaig, O. Ormandjiva, and K. Wan, "Context-based security and privacy for healthcare iot," in *IEEE International Conference on Smart Internet of Things (SmartIoT)*, 2018, pp. 122–128.

193. N. Madaan, M. A. Ahad, and S. M. Sastry, "Data integration in iot ecosystem: Information linkage as a privacy threat," *Computer Law & Security Review*, vol. 34, no. 1, pp. 125–133, 2018.

194. M. Dhiman, N. Gupta, U. Gupta, and Y. Kumar, "Lattice cryptography based geo-encrypted contact tracing for infection detection," 2021.

195. P. Kumar and L. Chouhan, "A privacy and session key based authentication scheme for medical iot networks," *Computer Communications*, vol. 166, pp. 154–164, 2021.

196. M. Almulhim and N. Zaman, "Proposing secure and lightweight authentication scheme for iot based e-health applications," in *20th IEEE International Conference on Advanced CommunicationTechnology (ICACT)*, 2018, pp. 481–487.

197. Y. Yang, X. Zheng, W. Guo, X. Liu, and V. Chang, "Privacy-preserving smart iot-based healthcare big data storage and self-adaptive access control system," *Information Sciences*, vol. 479, pp. 567–592, 2019.

198. E. Luo, M. Z. A. Bhuiyan, G. Wang, M. A. Rahman, J. Wu, and M. Atiquzzaman, "Privacyprotector: Privacy-protected patient data collection in iot-based healthcare systems," *IEEE Communications Magazine*, vol. 56, no. 2, pp. 163–168, 2018.

199. R. Hamza, Z. Yan, K. Muhammad, P. Bellavista, and F. Titouna, "A privacy-preserving cryptosystem for iot e-healthcare," *Information Sciences*, vol. 527, pp. 493–510, 2020.

200. A. Ibaida, A. Abuadbba, and N. Chilamkurti, "Privacy-preserving compression model for efficient iomt ecg sharing," *Computer Communications*, vol. 166, pp. 1–8, 2021.

201. R. Attarian and S. Hashemi, "An anonymity communication protocol for security and privacy of clients in iot-based mobile health transactions," *Computer Networks*, vol. 190, p. 107976, 2021.

202. J. A. Alzubi, "Blockchain-based lamport merkle digital signature: Authentication tool in iot healthcare," *Computer Communications*, vol. 170, pp. 200–208, 2021.

203. R. A. Mishra, A. Kalla, A. Braeken, and M. Liyanage, "Privacy protected blockchain based architecture and implementation for sharing of students' credentials," *Information Processing & Management*, vol. 58, no. 3, p. 102512, 2021.

204. W. Shao, C. Jia, Y. Xu, K. Qiu, Y. Gao, and Y. He, "Attrichain: Decentralized traceable anonymous identities in privacy-preserving permissioned blockchain," *Computers & Security*, vol. 99, p. 102069, 2020.

205. J. B. Bernabe, M. David, R. T. Moreno, J. P. Cordero, S. Bahloul, and A. Skarmeta, "Aries: Evaluation of a reliable and privacy-preserving european identity management framework," *Future Generation Computer Systems*, vol. 102, pp. 409–425, 2020.

206. S. Wood, "Adhering to privacy by design with identity-as-a-service," *Network Security*, vol. 2020, no. 7, pp. 14–17, 2020.

207. M. Gruteser and D. Grunwald, "Enhancing location privacy in wireless lan through disposable interface identifiers: A quantitative analysis," *Mobile Networks and Applications*, vol. 10, no. 3, pp. 315–325, 2005.

208. A. Fasbender, D. Kesdogan, and O. Kubitz, "Variable and scalable security: Protection of location information in mobile ip," in *Proceedings of Vehicular Technology Conference-VTC*, vol. 2, 1996, pp. 963–967.

209. I. Memon, "Authentication user's privacy: An integrating location privacy protection algorithm for secure moving objects in location based services," *Wireless Personal Communications*, vol. 82, no. 3, pp. 1585–1600, 2015.

210. K. Fawaz and K. G. Shin, "Location privacy protection for smartphone users," in *Proceedings of the 2014 ACM SIGSAC Conference on Computer and Communications Security*, 2014, pp. 239–250.

211. M. Han, L. Li, Y. Xie, J. Wang, Z. Duan, J. Li, and M. Yan, "Cognitive approach for location privacy protection," *IEEE Access*, vol. 6, pp. 13 466–13 477, 2018.

212. C. A. Ardagna, M. Cremonini, E. Damiani, S. D. C. Di Vimercati, and P. Samarati, "Location privacy protection through obfuscation-based techniques," in *IFIP Annual Conference on Data and Applications Security and Privacy*. Springer, 2007, pp. 47–60.

213. S. M. Randall, A. M. Ferrante, J. H. Boyd, J. K. Bauer, and J. B. Semmens, "Privacy-preserving record linkage on large real world datasets," *Journal of Biomedical Informatics*, vol. 50, pp. 205–212, 2014.

214. D. Hoare, A. Bussooa, S. Neale, N. Mirzai, and J. Mercer, "The future of cardiovascular stents: Bioresorbable and integrated biosensor technology," *Advanced Science*, vol. 6, no. 20, p. 1900856, 2019.

215. D. Vatsalan, P. Christen, and V. S. Verykios, "A taxonomy of privacy-preserving record linkage techniques," *Information Systems*, vol. 38, no. 6, pp. 946–969, 2013.

216. C.-Y. Chow, M. F. Mokbel, and W. G. Aref, "Casper* query processing for location services without compromising privacy," *ACM Transactions on Database Systems (TODS)*, vol. 34, no. 4, pp. 1–48, 2009.

217. G. Yubin, Z. Liankuan, L. Fengren, and L. Ximing, "A solution for privacy-preserving data manipulation and query on nosql database," *Journal of Computers*, vol. 8, no. 6, pp. 1427–1432, 2013.

218. N. I. Yekta and R. Lu, "Xrquery: Achieving communication-efficient privacy-preserving query for fog-enhanced iot," in *IEEE International Conference on Communications (ICC)*, 2018, pp. 1–6.

219. A. Nawaz, J. Peña Queralta, J. Guan, M. Awais, T. N. Gia, A. K. Bashir, H. Kan, and T. Westerlund, "Edge computing to secure iot data ownership and trade with the ethereum blockchain," *Sensors*, vol. 20, no. 14, p. 3965, 2020.

220. J.-H. Lee and H. Kim, "Security and privacy challenges in the internet of things [security and privacy matters]," *IEEE Consumer Electronics Magazine*, vol. 6, no. 3, pp. 134–136, 2017.

221. S. R. Department, "Global digital health market size 2019-2025 forecast," https://www.statista.com/statistics/1092869/global-digital-health-market-size-forecast/, Jun. 2021.

222. H. Jahankhani and J. Ibarra, "Digital forensic investigation for the internet of medical things (iomt)," *Forensic Legislative and Investigative Science*, vol. 5, no. 2, p. 029, 2019.

223. H. Mshali, T. Lemlouma, M. Moloney, and D. Magoni, "A survey on health monitoring systems for health smart homes," *International Journal of Industrial Ergonomics*, vol. 66, pp. 26–56, 2018.

224. "OWASP Internet of Things Project - OWASP," https://wiki.owasp.org/index.php/ OWASP Internet of Things Project, [Online; accessed 2021-08-19].

225. W. Zhou, Y. Jia, Y. Yao, L. Zhu, L. Guan, Y. Mao, P. Liu, and Y. Zhang, "Discovering and understanding the security hazards in the interactions between IoT devices, mobile apps, and clouds on smart home platforms," in *28th {USENIX} Security Symposium ({USENIX} Security 19)*, 2019, pp. 1133–1150.

226. S. Babar, P. Mahalle, A. Stango, N. Prasad, and R. Prasad, "Proposed security model and threat taxonomy for the internet of things (iot)," in *International Conference on Network Security and Applications*. Springer, 2010, pp. 420–429.

227. Y. Zhang, P. Xia, J. Luo, Z. Ling, B. Liu, and X. Fu, "Fingerprint attack against touch-enabled devices," in *Proceedings of the Second ACM Workshop on Security and Privacy in Smartphones and Mobile Devices*, 2012, pp. 57–68.

228. Q. Yue, Z. Ling, X. Fu, B. Liu, K. Ren, and W. Zhao, "Blind recognition of touched keys on mobile devices," in *Proceedings of the 2014 ACM SIGSAC Conference on Computer and Communications Security*, 2014, pp. 1403–1414.

229. S. S. Rani, J. A. Alzubi, S. Lakshmanaprabu, D. Gupta, and R. Manikandan, "Optimal users based secure data transmission on the internet of healthcare things (ioht) with lightweight block ciphers," *Multimedia Tools and Applications*, vol. 79, no. 47, pp. 35 405–35 424, 2020.

230. S. Vasile, D. Oswald, and T. Chothia, "Breaking all the things—a systematic survey of firmware extraction techniques for iot devices," in *International Conference on Smart Card Research and Advanced Applications*. Springer, 2018, pp. 171–185.

231. "IoT Attack Surface Areas," https://wiki.owasp.org/index.php/OWASP Internet of Things Project#tab=IoT Attack Surface Areas, [Online; accessed 2021-08-19].

232. M. Imdad, D. W. Jacob, H. Mahdin, Z. Baharum, S. M. Shaharudin, and M. S. Azmi, "Internet of things (iot); security requirements, attacks and counter measures," *Indonesian Journal of Electrical Engineering and Computer Science*, vol. 18, no. 3, pp. 1520–1530, 2020.

233. A. Tabassum, A. Erbad, A. Mohamed, and M. Guizani, "Privacy-preserving distributed IDS using incremental learning for IoT health systems," *IEEE Access*, vol. 9, pp. 14 271–14 283, 2021.

234. G. Thamilarasu, A. Odesile, and A. Hoang, "An intrusion detection system for internet of medical things," *IEEE Access*, vol. 8, pp. 181 560–181 576, 2020.

235. A. A. Hady, A. Ghubaish, T. Salman, D. Unal, and R. Jain, "Intrusion detection system for healthcare systems using medical and network data: A comparison study," *IEEE Access*, vol. 8, pp. 106 576–106 584, 2020.

236. H. Wu, H. Han, X. Wang, and S. Sun, "Research on artificial intelligence enhancing internet of things security: A survey," *IEEE Access*, vol. 8, pp. 153 826–153 848, 2020.

237. M. A. Rahman, M. S. Hossain, A. J. Showail, N. A. Alrajeh, and M. F. Alhamid, "A secure, private, and explainable ioht framework to support sustainable health monitoring in a smart city," *Sustainable Cities and Society*, vol. 72, p. 103083, 2021. [Online]. Available: https://www.sciencedirect.com/science/article/pii/S221067072100367X

238. M. Ahmed, S. Byreddy, A. Nutakki, L. F. Sikos, and P. Haskell-Dowland, "Ecu-ioht: A dataset for analyzing cyberattacks in internet of health things," *Ad Hoc Networks*, vol. 122, p. 102621, 2021. [Online]. Available: https://www.sciencedirect.com/science/article/pii/S1570870521001475

239. M. Stoyanova, Y. Nikoloudakis, S. Panagiotakis, E. Pallis, and E. K. Markakis, "A survey on the internet of things (iot) forensics: Challenges, approaches, and open issues," *IEEE Communications Surveys Tutorials*, vol. 22, no. 2, pp. 1191–1221, 2020.

240. "ISO/IEC 27043:2015 Information technology — Security techniques — Incident investigation principles and processes," https://www.iso.org/standard/44407.html, [Online; accessed 2021-08-19].

241. S. Zawoad and R. Hasan, "Faiot: Towards building a forensics aware eco system for the internet of things," in *2015 IEEE International Conference on Services Computing*, 2015, pp. 279–284.

242. L. Babun, A. K. Sikder, A. Acar, and A. S. Uluagac, "IoTDots: A digital forensics framework for smart environments." *CoRR*, vol. abs/1809.00745, 2018. [Online]. Available: http://dblp.uni-trier.de/db/journals/corr/corr1809.html#abs-1809-00745

243. "ISO/IEC 29100:2011 Information technology — Security techniques — Incident investigation principles and processes," https://www.iso.org/standard/45123.html, [Online; accessed 2021-08-19].

244. A. Nieto, R. Rios, and J. Lopez, "IoT-Forensics Meets Privacy: Towards Cooperative Digital Investigations," *Sensors*, vol. 18, no. 2, 2018. [Online]. Available: https://www.mdpi.com/1424-8220/18/2/492

245. A. Nieto, R. Roman, and J. Lopez, "Digital witness: Safeguarding digital evidence by using secure architectures in personal devices," *IEEE Network*, vol. 30, no. 6, pp. 34–41, 2016.

246. M. Hossain, Y. Karim, and R. Hasan, "Fif-iot: A forensic investigation framework for iot using a public digital ledger," in *IEEE International Congress on Internet of Things (ICIOT)*, 2018, pp. 33–40.

247. D.-P. Le, H. Meng, L. Su, S. L. Yeo, and V. Thing, "Biff: A blockchain-based iot forensics framework with identity privacy," in *TENCON 2018 - 2018 IEEE Region 10 Conference*, 2018, pp. 2372–2377.

248. Z. Tian, M. Li, M. Qiu, Y. Sun, and S. Su, "Block-def: A secure digital evidence framework using blockchain," *Information Sciences*, vol. 491, pp. 151–165, 2019. [Online]. Available: https://www.sciencedirect.com/science/article/pii/S002002551930297X

249. J. H. Ryu, P. K. Sharma, J. H. Jo, and J. H. Park, "A blockchain-based decentralized efficient investigation framework for iot digital forensics," *The Journal of Supercomputing*, vol. 75, no. 8, pp. 4372–4387, 2019.

250. M. M. Hossain, R. Hasan, and S. Zawoad, "Probe-iot: A public digital ledger based forensic investigation framework for iot." in *INFOCOM Workshops*, 2018, pp. 1–2.

251. L. Caviglione, S. Wendzel, and W. Mazurczyk, "The future of digital forensics: Challenges and the road ahead," *IEEE Security Privacy*, vol. 15, no. 6, pp. 12–17, 2017.

252. F. Kandah, Y. Singh, and C. Wang, "Colluding injected attack in mobile ad-hoc networks," in *IEEE Conference on Computer Communications Workshops (INFOCOM WKSHPS)*, 2011, pp. 235–240.

253. "OpenOCD: The open On-Chip Debugger," https://openocd.org/, [Online; accessed 2021-08-19].

254. A. Castro and A. Perez-Pons, "Virtual assistant for forensics recovery of iot devices," in *2021 7th IEEE International Conference on Big Data Security on Cloud (BigDataSecurity), IEEE International Conference on High Performance and Smart Computing, (HPSC) and IEEE International Conference on Intelligent Data and Security (IDS)*, 2021, pp. 186–190.

255. V. Ndatinya, Z. Xiao, V. R. Manepalli, K. Meng, and Y. Xiao, "Network forensics analysis using wireshark," *International Journal of Security and Networks*, vol. 10, no. 2, pp. 91–106, 2015.

256. S. Qureshi, S. Tunio, F. Akhtar, A. Wajahat, A. Nazir, and F. Ullah, "Network forensics: A comprehensive review of tools and techniques," *Network*, vol. 12, no. 5, 2021.

257. U. Lamping and E. Warnicke, "Wireshark user's guide," *Interface*, vol. 4, no. 6, p. 1, 2004.

258. M. Bettayeb, O. A. Waraga, M. A. Talib, Q. Nasir, and O. Einea, "Iot testbed security: Smart socket and smart thermostat," in *2019 IEEE Conference on Application, Information and Network Security (AINS)*, 2019, pp. 18–23.

259. "VirusTotal," https://www.virustotal.com, [Online; accessed 2021-08-19].

260. "The Exploit Database," https://www.exploit-db.com/, [Online; accessed 2021-08-19].

261. W. Jo, Y. Shin, H. Kim, D. Yoo, D. Kim, C. Kang, J. Jin, J. Oh, B. Na, and T. Shon, "Digital forensic practices and methodologies for AI speaker ecosystems," *Digital Investigation*, vol. 29, pp. S80–S93, 2019.

262. M.-A. Youn, Y. Lim, K. Seo, H. Chung, and S. Lee, "Forensic analysis for AI speaker with Display Echo Show 2nd generation as a case study," *Digital Investigation*, 2021.

263. B. Casey, "IoT crimes," https://cybersecurityventures.com/internet-of-things-hacks/, [Online; accessed 2021-08-19].

264. Z. Zorz, "Hacking smart plugs to enter business networks," https://www.helpnetsecurity.com/2018/08/23/hacking-smart-plugs/, [Online; accessed 2021-08-19].

265. A. Iqbal, J. Olegård, R. Ghimire, S. Jamshir, and A. Shalaginov, "Smart home forensics: An exploratory study on smart plug forensic analysis," in *2020 IEEE International Conference on Big Data (Big Data)*, 2020, pp. 2283–2290.

266. S. Vargas, "Privacy issues and digital forensic analysis for smart personal assistants," Ph.D. dissertation, Auckland University of Technology, 2020.

267. C. Krueger and S. McKeown, "Using amazon alexa apis as a source of digital evidence," in *2020 International Conference on Cyber Security and Protection of Digital Services (Cyber Security)*, 2020, pp. 1–8.

268. I. Yildirim, E. Bostanci, and M. S. Guzel, "Forensic analysis with anti-forensic case studies on amazon alexa and google assistant build-in smart home speakers," in *4th IEEE International Conference on Computer Science and Engineering (UBMK)*, 2019, pp. 1–3.

269. N. Scheidt and M. Adda, "Identification of iot devices for forensic investigation," in *2020 IEEE 10th International Conference on Intelligent Systems (IS)*, 2020, pp. 165–170.

270. S. Kim, M. Park, S. Lee, and J. Kim, "Smart home forensics—data analysis of iot devices," *Electronics*, vol. 9, no. 8, p. 1215, 2020.

271. W. Meng, Y. Cai, L. T. Yang, and W.-Y. Chiu, "Hybrid emotion-aware monitoring system based on brainwaves for internet of medical things," *IEEE Internet of Things Journal*, vol. 8, pp. 16014–16022, 2021.

272. K. S. Awaisi, S. Hussain, M. Ahmed, A. A. Khan, and G. Ahmed, "Leveraging iot and fog computing in healthcare systems," *IEEE Internet of Things Magazine*, vol. 3, no. 2, pp. 52–56, 2020.

273. W.-L. Chin, C.-C. Chang, C.-L. Tseng, Y.-Z. Huang, and T. Jiang, "Bayesian real-time qrs complex detector for healthcare system," *IEEE Internet of Things Journal*, vol. 6, no. 3, pp. 5540–5549, 2019.

274. M. N. Bhuiyan, M. M. Rahman, M. M. Billah, and D. Saha, "Internet of things (iot): A review of its enabling technologies in healthcare applications, standards protocols, security and market opportunities," *IEEE Internet of Things Journal*, 2021.

275. A. Ghubaish, T. Salman, M. Zolanvari, D. Unal, A. K. Al-Ali, and R. Jain, "Recent advances in the internet of medical things (iomt) systems security," *IEEE Internet of Things Journal*, vol. 8, pp. 8707–8718, 2020.

276. A. Algarni, "A survey and classification of security and privacy research in smart healthcare systems," *IEEE Access*, vol. 7, pp. 101 879–101 894, 2019.

277. T. Alladi, V. Chamola *et al.*, "Harci: A two-way authentication protocol for three entity healthcare iot networks," *IEEE Journal on Selected Areas in Communications*, vol. 39, no. 2, pp. 361–369, 2020.

278. L. Xu, X. Zhou, Y. Tao, L. Liu, X. Yu, and N. Kumar, "Intelligent security performance prediction for iot-enabled healthcare networks using improved cnn," *IEEE Transactions on Industrial Informatics*, 2021.

279. H. Tao, M. Z. A. Bhuiyan, A. N. Abdalla, M. M. Hassan, J. M. Zain, and T. Hayajneh, "Secured data collection with hardware-based ciphers for iot-based healthcare," *IEEE Internet of Things Journal*, vol. 6, no. 1, pp. 410–420, 2018.

280. W. Tang, J. Ren, K. Deng, and Y. Zhang, "Secure data aggregation of lightweight e-healthcare iot devices with fair incentives," *IEEE Internet of Things Journal*, vol. 6, no. 5, pp. 8714–8726, 2019.

281. R. Ding, H. Zhong, J. Ma, X. Liu, and J. Ning, "Lightweight privacy-preserving identity-based verifiable iot-based health storage system," *IEEE Internet of Things Journal*, vol. 6, no. 5, pp. 8393–8405, 2019.

282. D. He, R. Ye, S. Chan, M. Guizani, and Y. Xu, "Privacy in the internet of things for smart healthcare," *IEEE Communications Magazine*, vol. 56, no. 4, pp. 38–44, 2018.

283. L. Wang, Y. Ali, S. Nazir, and M. Niazi, "Isa evaluation framework for security of internet of health things system using ahp-topsis methods," *IEEE Access*, vol. 8, pp. 152 316–152 332, 2020.

284. A. Islam and S. Y. Shin, "A blockchain-based secure healthcare scheme with the assistance of unmanned aerial vehicle in internet of things," *Computers & Electrical Engineering*, vol. 84, p. 106627, 2020.

285. N. Tsafack, S. Sankar, B. Abd-El-Atty, J. Kengne, K. Jithin, A. Belazi, I. Mehmood, A. K. Bashir, O.-Y. Song, and A. A. Abd El-Latif, "A new chaotic map with dynamic analysis and encryption application in internet of health things," *IEEE Access*, vol. 8, pp. 137 731–137 744, 2020.

286. K. A. Awan, I. U. Din, A. Almogren, H. Almajed, I. Mohiuddin, and M. Guizani, "Neurotrust-artificial neural network-based intelligent trust management mechanism for large-scale internet of medical things," *IEEE Internet of Things Journal*, vol. 8, pp. 15672–15682, 2020.

287. J. Liu, L. Wang, and Y. Yu, "Improved security of a pairing-free certificateless aggregate signature in healthcare wireless medical sensor networks," *IEEE Internet of Things Journal*, vol. 7, no. 6, pp. 5256–5266, 2020.

288. B. D. Deebak and F. Al-Turjman, "Smart mutual authentication protocol for cloud based medical healthcare systems using internet of medical things," *IEEE Journal on Selected Areas in Communications*, vol. 39, no. 2, pp. 346–360, 2020.

289. Y. Zhang, D. He, M. S. Obaidat, P. Vijayakumar, and K.-F. Hsiao, "Efficient identity-based distributed decryption scheme for electronic personal health record sharing system," *IEEE Journal on Selected Areas in Communications*, vol. 39, no. 2, pp. 384–395, 2020.

290. Z. Wang, "Blind batch encryption-based protocol for secure and privacy-preserving medical services in smart connected health," *IEEE Internet of Things Journal*, vol. 6, no. 6, pp. 9555–9562, 2019.

291. X. Li, J. Peng, M. S. Obaidat, F. Wu, M. K. Khan, and C. Chen, "A secure three-factor user authentication protocol with forward secrecy for wireless medical sensor network systems," *IEEE Systems Journal*, vol. 14, no. 1, pp. 39–50, 2019.

292. W. Meng, W. Li, and L. Zhu, "Enhancing medical smartphone networks via blockchain-based trust management against insider attacks," *IEEE Transactions on Engineering Management*, vol. 67, no. 4, pp. 1377–1386, 2019.

293. Y. Meng, Z. Huang, G. Shen, and C. Ke, "Sdn-based security enforcement framework for data sharing systems of smart healthcare," *IEEE Transactions on Network and Service Management*, vol. 17, no. 1, pp. 308–318, 2019.

294. A. Krall, D. Finke, and H. Yang, "Mosaic privacy-preserving mechanisms for healthcare analytics," *IEEE Journal of Biomedical and Health Informatics*, vol. 25, no. 6, pp. 2184–2192, 2020.

295. L. Fang, Y. Li, Z. Liu, C. Yin, M. Li, and Z. J. Cao, "A practical model based on anomaly detection for protecting medical iot control services against external attacks," *IEEE Transactions on Industrial Informatics*, vol. 17, no. 6, pp. 4260–4269, 2020.

296. F. Rezaeibagha, Y. Mu, K. Huang, and L. Chen, "Secure and efficient data aggregation for iot monitoring systems," *IEEE Internet of Things Journal*, vol. 8, no. 10, pp. 8056–8063, 2020.

297. M. H. Chinaei, H. H. Gharakheili, and V. Sivaraman, "Optimal witnessing of healthcare iot data using blockchain logging contract," *IEEE Internet of Things Journal*, vol. 8, pp. 10117–10130, 2021.

298. Y. Sun, J. Liu, K. Yu, M. Alazab, and K. Lin, "Pmrss: Privacy-preserving medical record searching scheme for intelligent diagnosis in iot healthcare," *IEEE Transactions on Industrial Informatics*, 2021.

299. M. A. Jan, F. Khan, S. Mastorakis, M. Adil, A. Akbar, and N. Stergiou, "Lightiot: Lightweight and secure communication for energy-efficient iot in health informatics," *IEEE Transactions on Green Communications and Networking*, 2021.

300. M. Masud, G. S. Gaba, K. Choudhary, M. S. Hossain, M. F. Alhamid, and G. Muhammad, "Lightweight and anonymity-preserving user authentication scheme for iot-based healthcare," *IEEE Internet of Things Journal*, 2021.

301. F. Alshehri and G. Muhammad, "A comprehensive survey of the internet of things (iot) and ai-based smart healthcare." *IEEE Access*, vol. 9, no. January, pp. 3660–3678, 2021.

302. Y. A. Qadri, A. Nauman, Y. B. Zikria, A. V. Vasilakos, and S. W. Kim, "The future of healthcare internet of things: A survey of emerging technologies," *IEEE Communications Surveys & Tutorials*, vol. 22, no. 2, pp. 1121–1167, 2020.

303. Z. Yang, B. Liang, and W. Ji, "An intelligent end-edge-cloud architecture for visual iot assisted healthcare systems," *IEEE Internet of Things Journal*, vol. 8, pp. 16779–16786, 2021.

304. H. Habibzadeh, K. Dinesh, O. R. Shishvan, A. Boggio-Dandry, G. Sharma, and T. Soy-
     ata, "A survey of healthcare internet of things (hiot): A clinical perspective," *IEEE
     Internet of Things Journal*, vol. 7, no. 1, pp. 53–71, 2019.

305. M. Kumar and S. Chand, "A secure and efficient cloud-centric internet-of-medical-
     things-enabled smart healthcare system with public verifiability," *IEEE Internet of
     Things Journal*, vol. 7, no. 10, pp. 10 650–10 659, 2020.

306. B. S. Egala, A. K. Pradhan, V. R. Badarla, and S. P. Mohanty, "Fortified-chain: A
     blockchain based framework for security and privacy assured internet of medical things
     with effective access control," *IEEE Internet of Things Journal*, vol. 8, pp. 11717–
     11731, 2021.

307. S. B. Baker, W. Xiang, and I. Atkinson, "Internet of things for smart healthcare: Tech-
     nologies, challenges, and opportunities," *IEEE Access*, vol. 5, pp. 26 521–26 544, 2017.

308. S. Popli, R. K. Jha, and S. Jain, "A survey on energy efficient narrowband internet
     of things (nbiot): Architecture, application and challenges," *IEEE Access*, vol. 7, pp.
     16 739–16 776, 2018.

309. Ericsson, "Transforming healthcare with 5g," https://www.ericsson.com/en/cases/
     2016/5gtuscany/transforming-healthcare-with-5g, accessed: 2021-11-11.

310. S. India, "Healthcare iot solutions," https://www.se.com/in/en/work/solutions/
     for-business/healthcare/, accessed: 2021-11-11.

311. Viz.ai, "A.i. powered synchronized stroke care," https://www.viz.ai/ischemic-stroke,
     accessed: 2021-11-1.

312. P. India, "Reimagining the possible in the indian healthcare ecosystem with emerging
     technologies," https://www.pwc.in/industries/healthcare/reimagining-the-possible-in-
     the-indian-healthcare-ecosystem//-with-emerging-technologies.html, accessed: 2021-
     11-21.

313. S. Labs, "Smart e-health gateway," https://www.skyfilabs.com/project-ideas/
     smart-e-health-gateway, accessed: 2021-10-11.

314. Nokia, "Private network solutions for real-time healthcare and the cloud," https://www.
     nokia.com/networks/industries/healthcare/, accessed: 2021-10-11.

315. SARAS, "Smart autonomous robotic assistant surgeon," https://saras-project.eu/, ac-
     cessed: 2021-10-11.

316. Medtronic, "Medtronic-robotic assisted surgery," https://www.medtronic.com/
     covidien/en-gb/robotic-assisted-surgery/hugo-ras-system.html, accessed: 2021-10-
     11.

317. D. Magician, "To develop a lightweight intelligent robotic arm," https://www.dobot.cc/
     dobot-magician/product-overview.html?gclid=CjwKCAjwtpGGBhBJEiwAyRZX2n
     8l3Wec7bt//I9Dh7HZef6cLce63kcemgBp7CKb7SaazBXQ-aTI4HZRoCFJEQAvD˙
     BwE, accessed: 2021-10-11.

318. D. Yu, L. Zhang, Y. Chen, Y. Ma, and J. Chen, "Large-scale iot devices firmware identification based on weak password," *IEEE Access*, vol. 8, pp. 7981–7992, 2020.

319. W. Han, Z. Li, M. Ni, G. Gu, and W. Xu, "Shadow attacks based on password reuses: A quantitative empirical analysis," *IEEE Transactions on Dependable and Secure Computing*, vol. 15, no. 2, pp. 309–320, 2016.

320. P. Anand, Y. Singh, A. Selwal, M. Alazab, S. Tanwar, and N. Kumar, "Iot vulnerability assessment for sustainable computing: Threats, current solutions, and open challenges," *IEEE Access*, vol. 8, pp. 168 825–168 853, 2020.

321. X. Liu, C. Qian, W. G. Hatcher, H. Xu, W. Liao, and W. Yu, "Secure internet of things (iot)-based smart-world critical infrastructures: Survey, case study and research opportunities," *IEEE Access*, vol. 7, pp. 79 523–79 544, 2019.

322. N. Mishra and S. Pandya, "Internet of things applications, security challenges, attacks, intrusion detection, and future visions: A systematic review," *IEEE Access*, 2021.

323. "Reimagining patient-centric clinical trials with the iomt," https://www.iconplc.com/insights/patient-centricity/reimagining-patient-centricity-with-the-iomt/, accessed: 2021-07-31.

324. Q. Qi, X. Chen, C. Zhong, and Z. Zhang, "Integrated sensing, computation and communication in b5g cellular internet of things," *IEEE Transactions on Wireless Communications*, vol. 20, no. 1, pp. 332–344, 2020.

325. S. Forrest, K. Baker, and M. Ketel, "Internet of medical things: Enabling key technologies," in *SoutheastCon 2021*. IEEE, 2021, pp. 1–5.

326. J. D. Trigo, H. Klaina, I. P. Guembe, P. Lopez-Iturri, J. J. Astrain, A. V. Alejos, F. Falcone, and L. Serrano-Arriezu, "Patient tracking in a multi-building, tunnel-connected hospital complex," *IEEE Sensors Journal*, vol. 20, no. 23, pp. 14 453–14 464, 2020.

327. B. Qian, H. Zhou, T. Ma, K. Yu, Q. Yu, and X. Shen, "Multi-operator spectrum sharing for massive iot coexisting in 5g/b5g wireless networks," *IEEE Journal on Selected Areas in Communications*, vol. 39, no. 3, pp. 881–895, 2020.

328. S. Sakib, T. Tazrin, M. M. Fouda, Z. M. Fadlullah, and N. Nasser, "An efficient and lightweight predictive channel assignment scheme for multiband b5g-enabled massive iot: A deep learning approach," *IEEE Internet of Things Journal*, vol. 8, no. 7, pp. 5285–5297, 2020.

329. X. Chen, D. W. K. Ng, W. Yu, E. G. Larsson, N. Al-Dhahir, and R. Schober, "Massive access for 5g and beyond," *IEEE Journal on Selected Areas in Communications*, vol. 39, no. 3, pp. 615–637, 2020.

330. P. S. Hall and Y. Hao, *Antennas and Propagation for Body-centric Wireless Communications*. Artech House, 2012.

331. J. Wang and Q. Wang, *Body Body Area Communications: Channel Modeling, Communication Systems, and EMC*. John Wiley & Sons, 2012.

332. M. U. A. Siddiqui, F. Qamar, F. Ahmed, Q. N. Nguyen, and R. Hassan, "Interference management in 5g and beyond network: Requirements, challenges and future directions," *IEEE Access*, vol. 9, pp. 68 932–68 965, 2021.

333. Z. Shelby, K. Hartke, C. Bormann, and B. Frank, "Constrained application protocol (coap). draft-ietfcore-coap-12," 2012.

334. K. Jia, J. Xiao, S. Fan, and G. He, "A mqtt/mqtt-sn-based user energy management system for automated residential demand response: Formal verification and cyber-physical performance evaluation," *Applied Sciences*, vol. 8, no. 7, p. 1035, 2018.

335. D. P. Isravel, S. Silas *et al.*, "A comprehensive review on the emerging iot-cloud based technologies for smart healthcare," in *2020 6th International Conference on Advanced Computing and Communication Systems (ICACCS)*. IEEE, 2020, pp. 606–611.

336. R. Hegde, S. Ranjana, and C. Divya, "Survey on development of smart healthcare monitoring system in iot environment," in *2021 5th International Conference on Computing Methodologies and Communication (ICCMC)*. IEEE, 2021, pp. 395–399.

337. S. K. Routray and S. Anand, "Narrowband iot for healthcare," in *2017 International Conference on Information Communication and Embedded Systems (ICICES)*. IEEE, 2017, pp. 1–4.

338. S. Anand and S. K. Routray, "Issues and challenges in healthcare narrowband iot," in *2017 International Conference on Inventive Communication and Computational Technologies (ICICCT)*. IEEE, 2017, pp. 486–489.

339. M. Suguna, M. Ramalakshmi, J. Cynthia, and D. Prakash, "A survey on cloud and internet of things based healthcare diagnosis," in *2018 4th International Conference on Computing Communication and Automation (ICCCA)*. IEEE, 2018, pp. 1–4.

340. Y. Shi, G. Ding, H. Wang, H. E. Roman, and S. Lu, "The fog computing service for healthcare," in *2015 2nd International Symposium on Future Information and Communication Technologies for Ubiquitous HealthCare (Ubi-HealthTech)*. IEEE, 2015, pp. 1–5.

341. O. Bibani, C. Mouradian, S. Yangui, R. H. Glitho, W. Gaaloul, N. B. Hadj-Alouane, M. Morrow, and P. Polakos, "A demo of iot healthcare application provisioning in hybrid cloud/fog environment," in *2016 IEEE International Conference on Cloud Computing Technology and Science (CloudCom)*. IEEE, 2016, pp. 472–475.

342. S. El Kafhali, K. Salah, and S. B. Alla, "Performance evaluation of iot-fog-cloud deployment for healthcare services," in *2018 4th International Conference on Cloud Computing Technologies and Applications (Cloudtech)*. IEEE, 2018, pp. 1–6.

343. S. Ahmed, M. Saqib, M. Adil, T. Ali, and A. Ishtiaq, "Integration of cloud computing with internet of things and wireless body area network for effective healthcare," in *2017 International Symposium on Wireless Systems and Networks (ISWSN)*. IEEE, 2017, pp. 1–6.

344. P. Kanehanadevi, D. Selvapandian, L. Raja, and R. Dhanapal, "Cloud-based protection and performance improvement in the e-health management framework," in *2020 Fourth International Conference on I-SMAC (IoT in Social, Mobile, Analytics and Cloud)(I-SMAC)*. IEEE, 2020, pp. 268–270.

345. J. Hong, P. Morris, and J. Seo, "Interconnected personal health record ecosystem using iot cloud platform and hl7 fhir," in *2017 IEEE International Conference on Healthcare Informatics (ICHI)*. IEEE, 2017, pp. 362–367.

346. F. Sadoughi and L. Erfannia, "Health information system in a cloud computing context." in *eHealth*, 2017, pp. 290–297.

347. T. Karatekin, S. Sancak, G. Celik, S. Topcuoglu, G. Karatekin, P. Kirci, and A. Okatan, "Interpretable machine learning in healthcare through generalized additive model with pairwise interactions (ga2m): Predicting severe retinopathy of prematurity," in *2019 International Conference on Deep Learning and Machine Learning in Emerging Applications (Deep-ML)*. IEEE, 2019, pp. 61–66.

348. S. Durga, R. Nag, and E. Daniel, "Survey on machine learning and deep learning algorithms used in internet of things (iot) healthcare," in *3rd International Conference on Computing Methodologies and Communication (ICCMC)*, 2019, pp. 1018–1022.

349. K. Yazhini and D. Loganathan, "A state of art approaches on deep learning models in healthcare: An application perspective," in *2019 3rd International Conference on Trends in Electronics and Informatics (ICOEI)*. IEEE, 2019, pp. 195–200.

350. P. Sujatha and K. Mahalakshmi, "Performance evaluation of supervised machine learning algorithms in prediction of heart disease," in *2020 IEEE International Conference for Innovation in Technology (INOCON)*. IEEE, 2020, pp. 1–7.

351. V. Manimegalai, A. Gayathri, V. Mohanapriya, C. Gowtham, C. A. Kumar, and S. D. Kanna, "Spruce fitness observation method using iot and machine learning," in *2021 5th International Conference on Intelligent Computing and Control Systems (ICICCS)*. IEEE, 2021, pp. 384–388.

352. L. von Rueden, S. Mayer, K. Beckh, B. Georgiev, S. Giesselbach, R. Heese, B. Kirsch, J. Pfrommer, A. Pick, R. Ramamurthy *et al.*, "Informed machine learning–a taxonomy and survey of integrating knowledge into learning systems," *arXiv preprint arXiv:1903.12394*, 2019.

353. L. James, "Digital twins will revolutionise healthcare: Digital twin technology has the potential to transform healthcare in a variety of ways–improving the diagnosis and treatment of patients, streamlining preventative care and facilitating new approaches for hospital planning," *Engineering & Technology*, vol. 16, no. 2, pp. 50–53, 2021.

354. A. Ricci, A. Croatti, and S. Montagna, "Pervasive and connected digital twins–a vision for digital health," *IEEE Internet Computing*, 2021.

355. H. Elayan, M. Aloqaily, and M. Guizani, "Digital twin for intelligent context-aware iot healthcare systems," *IEEE Internet of Things Journal*, vol. 8, pp. 16749–16757, 2021.

356. N. Wickramasinghe, P. P. Jayaraman, J. Zelcer, A. R. M. Forkan, N. Ulapane, R. Kaul, and S. Vaughan, "A vision for leveraging the concept of digital twins to support the provision of personalised cancer care," *IEEE Internet Computing*, 2021.

357. R. Martinez-Velazquez, R. Gamez, and A. El Saddik, "Cardio twin: A digital twin of the human heart running on the edge," in *2019 IEEE International Symposium on Medical Measurements and Applications (MeMeA)*. IEEE, 2019, pp. 1–6.

358. S. Alromaihi, W. Elmedany, and C. Balakrishna, "Cyber security challenges of deploying iot in smart cities for healthcare applications," in *2018 6th International Conference on Future Internet of Things and Cloud Workshops (FiCloudW)*. IEEE, 2018, pp. 140–145.

359. S. A. Butt, J. L. Diaz-Martinez, T. Jamal, A. Ali, E. De-La-Hoz-Franco, and M. Shoaib, "Iot smart health security threats," in *2019 19th International Conference on Computational Science and Its Applications (ICCSA)*. IEEE, 2019, pp. 26–31.

360. M. A. Lawal, R. A. Shaikh, and S. R. Hassan, "A ddos attack mitigation framework for iot networks using fog computing," *Procedia Computer Science*, vol. 182, pp. 13–20, 2021.

361. L. Huraj, T. Horak, P. Strelec, and P. Tanuska, "Mitigation against ddos attacks on an iot-based production line using machine learning," *Applied Sciences*, vol. 11, no. 4, p. 1847, 2021.

362. C. Eken and H. Eken, "Security threats and recommendation in iot healthcare," in *Proceedings of The 9th EUROSIM Congress on Modelling and Simulation, EUROSIM 2016, The 57th SIMS Conference on Simulation and Modelling SIMS 2016*, no. 142. Linköping University Electronic Press, 2018, pp. 369–374.

363. R. Khadim, A. Ennaciri, M. Erritali, and A. Maaden, "Impact of location data freshness on routing in wireless sensor networks," in *Europe and MENA Cooperation Advances in Information and Communication Technologies*. Springer, 2017, pp. 373–382.

364. J. Andonegui, D. Aliseda, L. Serrano, A. Eguzkiza, N. Arruti, L. Arias, and A. Alcaine, "Evaluation of a telemedicine model to follow up patients with exudative age-related macular degeneration," *Retina*, vol. 36, no. 2, pp. 279–284, 2016.

365. Z. Xu, C. Xu, J. Xu, and X. Meng, "A computationally efficient authentication and key agreement scheme for multi-server switching in wban," *International Journal of Sensor Networks*, vol. 35, no. 3, pp. 143–160, 2021.

366. R. Punj and R. Kumar, "Technological aspects of wbans for health monitoring: A comprehensive review," *Wireless Networks*, vol. 25, no. 3, pp. 1–33, 2018.

367. S. P. Chatrati, G. Hossain, A. Goyal, A. Bhan, S. Bhattacharya, D. Gaurav, and S. M. Tiwari, "Smart home health monitoring system for predicting type 2 diabetes and hypertension," *Journal of King Saud University-Computer and Information Sciences*, vol. 34, pp. 862–870, 2020.

368. V. Palanisamy and R. Thirunavukarasu, "Implications of big data analytics in developing healthcare frameworks–a review," *Journal of King Saud University-Computer and Information Sciences*, vol. 31, no. 4, pp. 415–425, 2019.

369. M. E. Bayrakdar, "Fuzzy logic based coordinator node selection approach in wireless medical sensor networks," in *2019 4th International Conference on Computer Science and Engineering (UBMK)*, 2019, pp. 340–343.

370. R. Punj and R. Kumar, "Energy efficient dynamic cluster head and routing path selection strategy for wbans," *Wireless Personal Communications*, vol. 113, no. 1, pp. 1–26, 2020.

371. T. Munirathinam, S. Ganapathy, and A. Kannan, "Cloud and iot based privacy preserved e-healthcare system using secured storage algorithm and deep learning," *Journal of Intelligent & Fuzzy Systems*, vol. 39, no. 3, pp. 3011–3023, 2020.

372. U. Vijay and N. Gupta, "Clustering in wsn based on minimum spanning tree using divide and conquer approach," *International Journal of Computer and Information Engineering*, vol. 7, no. 7, pp. 926–930, 2013.

373. F. Castanedo, "A review of data fusion techniques," *The Scientific World Journal*, vol. 2013, pp. 1–19, 2013.

374. K. Zhang, X. Liang, M. Baura, R. Lu, and X. S. Shen, "PHDA: A priority based health data aggregation with privacy preservation for cloud assisted wbans," *Information Sciences*, vol. 284, pp. 130–141, 2014.

375. O. H. Salman, M. F. A. Rasid, M. I. Saripan, and S. K. Subramaniam, "Multi-sources data fusion framework for remote triage prioritization in telehealth," *Journal of Medical Systems*, vol. 38, no. 9, pp. 1–23, 2014.

376. A. K. Idrees, A. K. M. Al-Qurabat, C. Abou Jaoude, and W. L. Al-Yaseen, "Integrated divide and conquer with enhanced k-means technique for energy-saving data aggregation in wireless sensor networks," in *2019 15th International Wireless Communications & Mobile Computing Conference (IWCMC)*, 2019, pp. 973–978.

377. N. Kaur and S. Singh, "Optimized cost effective and energy efficient routing protocol for wireless body area networks," *Ad Hoc Networks*, vol. 61, pp. 65–84, 2017.

378. V. Navya and P. Deepalakshmi, "Energy efficient routing for critical physiological parameters in wireless body area networks under mobile emergency scenarios," *Computers & Electrical Engineering*, vol. 72, pp. 512–525, 2018.

379. A. Ullah, G. Said, M. Sher, and H. Ning, "Fog-assisted secure healthcare data aggregation scheme in iot-enabled wsn," *Peer-to-Peer Networking and Applications*, vol. 13, pp. 163–174, 2019.

380. S. Sirsikar and S. Anavatti, "Issues of data aggregation methods in wireless sensor network: A survey," *Procedia Computer Science*, vol. 49, pp. 194–201, 2015.

381. S. Misra and S. Chatterjee, "Social choice considerations in cloud-assisted wban architecture for post-disaster healthcare: Data aggregation and channelization," *Information Sciences*, vol. 284, pp. 95–117, 2014.

382. M. N. Halgamuge, M. Zukerman, K. Ramamohanarao, and H. L. Vu, "An estimation of sensor energy consumption," *Progress in Electromagnetics Research*, vol. 12, pp. 259–295, 2009.

383. W. R. Heinzelman, A. Chandrakasan, and H. Balakrishnan, "Energy-efficient communication protocol for wireless microsensor networks," in *Proceedings of the 33rd IEEE Annual Hawaii International Conference on System Sciences*, 2000, pp. 1–10.

384. N. Datta, *Study and Design of Energy Efficient Block Cipher for Wireless Body Area Networks (WBANs)*, Thesis, IISC Banglore, India, 2014.

385. F. Dubosson, J.-E. Ranvier, S. Bromuri, J.-P. Calbimonte, J. Ruiz, and M. Schumacher, "The open d1namo dataset: A multi-modal dataset for research on non-invasive type 1 diabetes management," *Informatics in Medicine Unlocked*, vol. 13, pp. 92–100, 2018.

386. S. Care, "Everything you wanted to know about smart health care," *IEEE Consumer and Electronics Magazine*, vol. 7, pp. 18–28, 2018.

387. S. Global, "White paper: The age of the smart hospital," 2020, https://new.siemens.com/global/en/products/buildings/contact/the-age-of-the-smart-hospital.html.

388. I. U. Din, A. Almogren, M. Guizani, and M. Zuair, "A decade of internet of things: Analysis in the light of healthcare applications," *IEEE Access*, vol. 7, pp. 89 967–89 979, 2019.

389. K. Vikas, B. Nils, S. Ulrica, and T. Johan, "Building the smart hospital agenda," January 2017, https://www.adlittle.com/sites/default/files/viewpoints/ADL˙Smart%20Hospital.pdf.

390. S. Tuli, S. Tuli, G. Wander, P. Wander, S. S. Gill, S. Dustdar, R. Sakellariou, and O. Rana, "Next generation technologies for smart healthcare: Challenges, vision, model, trends and future directions," *Internet Technology Letters*, vol. 3, no. 2, p. e145, 2020.

391. S. Tian, W. Yang, J. M. Le Grange, P. Wang, W. Huang, and Z. Ye, "Smart healthcare: Making medical care more intelligent," *Global Health Journal*, vol. 3, no. 3, pp. 62–65, 2019.

392. A. Fahmy, H. Altaf, A. Al Nabulsi, A. Al-Ali, and R. Aburukba, "Role of rfid technology in smart city applications," in *2019 International Conference on Communications, Signal Processing, and Their Applications (ICCSPA)*. IEEE, 2019, pp. 1–6.

393. M. G. Institute, "Smart cities: Digital solutions for a more livable future," June 2018, https://www.mckinsey.com/business-functions/operations/our-insights/smart-cities-digital-solutions-for-a-more-livable-future.

394. A. Ahad, M. Tahir, and K.-L. A. Yau, "5g-based smart healthcare network: Architecture, taxonomy, challenges and future research directions," *IEEE Access*, vol. 7, pp. 100 747–100 762, 2019.

395. S. U. Amin, M. S. Hossain, G. Muhammad, M. Alhussein, and M. A. Rahman, "Cognitive smart healthcare for pathology detection and monitoring," *IEEE Access*, vol. 7, pp. 10 745–10 753, 2019.

396. S. I. W. Paper, "Mount sinai hospital improves patient experience with mobile tech," May 2020, https://insights.samsung.com/2020/03/03/mount-sinai-hospital-improves-patient-experience-with\-mobile-technology/.

397. W. E. Forum, "Can ai predict which coronavirus patients will get the sickest?" May 2020, https://www.weforum.org/agenda/2020/05/we-designed-an-experimental-ai-tool-to-predict-which\-covid-19-patients-are-going-to-get-the-sickest.

398. "The official uk government website for data and insights on coronavirus covid-19," 2021, https://coronavirus.data.gov.uk/?˙ga=2.70409811.251160290.1600535149-223926311.1600535149.

399. "Coronavirus (covid-19) - google news," 2021, https://news.google.com/covid19/map? hl=en-IN&gl=IN&ceid=IN%3Aen.

400. "Covid-19 symptom check," 2021, https://c19check.com/terms-and-conditions.

401. Greenbiz, "Israel's 'smart commuting' shows what public transport could be like after covid-19," August 2020, https://www.greenbiz.com/article/israels-smart-commuting-shows-what-public-transport-could-be\-after-covid-19.

402. "U.k. scientists tap ai for better ventilation for covid patients - bloomberg," July 2020, https://www.bloomberg.com/news/articles/2020-07-21/u-k-scientists-tap-ai-for-better-ventilation-for-covid-patients.

403. Smarttampere, "Health and well-being," April 2020, https://smarttampere.fi/en/network/health-and-well-being/.

404. T. S. City, "Wear-free elderly people's safety detection and health management demonstration project," April 2019, https://smartcity.taipei/projdetail/8.

405. ——, "Smart urban and rural: Taipei city and lienjiang county telemedicine experimental project," October 2018, https://smartcity.taipei/projdetail/142.

406. "Smart city," 2021, https://smartcity.taipei/projects/0?lang=en.

407. P. P. Release, "Philips and dutch rijnstate hospital sign 10-year agreement to build a virtual hospital for large-scale connected care," May 2018, https://www.philips.com/a-w/about/news/archive/standard/news/press/2018/20180516-philips-and-dutch-rijnstate-hospital-sign\-10-year-agreement-to-build-a-virtual-hospital.html.

408. O. I. Report, "Dubai to deploy cutting-edge ai devices in healthcare," June 2020, https://insights.omnia-health.com/hospital-management/dubai-deploy-cutting-edge-ai-devices-healthcare.

409. "How singapore is working towards a healthier tomorrow smartly," March 2017, https://www.edb.gov.sg/en/news-and-events/insights/innovation/how-singapore-is-working-towards-a-healthier-tomorrow---smartly.html.

410. A. Oriel, "How artificial intelligence is helping to fight against coronavirus in india?" August 2020, https://www.analyticsinsight.net/artificial-intelligence-helping-fight-coronavirus-india/.

411. V. Kulkarni, "How india is using artificial intelligence to combat covid-19 - the week," July 2020, https://www.theweek.in/news/sci-tech/2020/07/31/how-india-is-using-artificial-intelligence-to-combat-covid-19.html?utm˙source=dlvr.it& utm˙medium=facebook.

412. R. Dillet, "French contact-tracing app stopcovid has been activated 1.8 million times but only sent 14 notifications," June 2020, https://techcrunch.com/2020/06/23/french-contact-tracing-app-stopcovid-has-been-activated-1-8\-million-times-but-only-sent-14-notifications/.

413. J. Vincent, "France is using ai to check whether people are wearing masks on public transport - the verge," May 2020, https://www.theverge.com/2020/5/7/21250357/ france-masks-public-transport-mandatory-ai\-surveillance-camera-software.

414. G. Adams, "Warthog ugv joins fight against covid-19 - clearpath robotics," August 2020, https://clearpathrobotics.com/blog/2020/08/warthog-ugv-joins-fight-against-covid-19/.

Index